P9-DKF-378

The Magic of Essential Oils

Aromatherapy offers something for nearly everyone: medical practitioners seeking natural treatments, massage therapists and other body workers looking for an effective form of plant energy to use in their work, psychologists who want a natural way to treat stress and other imbalances, the spiritual seeker on the path to enlightenment, or the person who uses lavender oil to give her environment a pleasing scent.

Essential oils have a magic that creates and promotes transformation in people's lives on many levels. They are highly concentrated forms of herbal energy that represent the soul, or life force, of the plant. When aromatic vapors are inhaled, they can influence areas of the brain inaccessible to conscious control, such as emotions and hormonal responses. Application of the oils in massage can enhance the benefits of body work on the muscular, lymphatic, and nervous systems. Cutaneous application of the oils helps to influence the main body systems.

All of these therapeutic uses of essential oils—the Earth's naturally healing nectars—increase harmony and balance. This comprehensive book provides all the knowledge you need to benefit from the many ways aromatherapy can bring balance into your life.

About the Author

Ann Berwick was born in Seattle, Washington and in 1970 moved with her family to England. She attended school in England and earned her B.S. in Sociology at the Polytechnic of North London. She currently lives with her family and dog outside Boulder, Colorado.

Ann has been involved in aromatherapy for more than a decade. She received her initial training with Patricia Davis at the London School of Aromatherapy and also trained with Shirley Price. In the mid-eighties she opened a holistic health clinic in suburban London. She returned to the United States in 1989 and started Quintessence Aromatherapy Inc., now called Ann Berwick Aromatherapy, which offers a certification program and Shirley Price products. Ann has written for and been featured in the local and national press, serves as a consultant for spas and companies, and maintains her own aromatherapy practice. As a founding member and former President of the National Association for Holistic Aromatherapy, Ann promotes training standards and public knowledge about the subject. She has studied reflexology, herbalism, flower essence therapy, and color therapy. She is also a licensed massage therapist and esthetician.

To Write to the Author

If you wish to contact the author or would like more information about this book, please write to the author in care Llewellyn Worldwide, and we will forward your request. Both the author and publisher appreciate hearing from you and learning of your enjoyment of this book and how it has helped you. Llewellyn Worldwide cannot guarantee that every letter written to the author can be answered, but all will be forwarded. Please write to:

Ann Berwick
c/o Llewellyn Worldwide
P.O. Box 64383-033, St. Paul, MN 55164-0383, U.S.A.

Please enclose a self-addressed, stamped envelope for reply, or $1.00 to cover costs. If outside the U.S.A., enclose international postal reply coupon.

Free Catalog from Llewellyn

For more than 90 years Llewellyn has brought its readers knowledge in the fields of metaphysics and human potential. Learn about the newest books in spiritual guidance, natural healing, astrology, occult philosophy, and more. Enjoy book reviews, new age articles, a calender of events, plus current products and services. To get your free copy of Llewellyn's New Worlds of Mind and Spirit, send your name and address to:

Llewellyn's New Worlds of Mind and Spirit
P.O. Box 64383-033, St. Paul, MN 55164-0383, U.S.A.

Holistic Aromatherapy

Balance the Body and Soul with Essential Oils

by Ann Berwick

1994
Llewellyn Publications
St. Paul, Minnesota 55164-0383, U.S.A.

Holistic Aromatherapy. Copyright © 1994 by Ann Berwick. All rights reserved. Printed in the United States of America. No part of this book may be used or reproduced in any manner whatsoever without written permission from Llewellyn Publications except in the case of brief quotations embodied in critical articles and reviews.

FIRST EDITION
First Printing, 1994

Cover design: Alexandra Lumen
Plant illustrations: June Zenner
Book design and layout: Michelle Dahn

Library of Congress Cataloging-in-Publication Data
Berwick, Ann, 1953–
    Holistic aromatherapy : balance the body and soul with essential oils / by Ann Berwick.
        p.   cm.
    Includes bibliographical references and index.
    ISBN 0-87542-033-8
    1. Aromatherapy.   I. Title.
RM666.A68B47   1994
615' .321--dc20   93-48571
                                                                  CIP

Llewellyn Publications
A Division of Llewellyn Worldwide, Ltd.
P.O. Box 64383, St. Paul, MN 55164-0383

Dedication

This book is dedicated to my parents, who have supported me in every situation, my husband Robert, and my children, Adam, Alex, and Natasha, who make it all worthwhile.

Special thanks are due to my father, whose patient and careful editing of my manuscript brought this book into being. It would not have happened without him.

Of course, I cannot forget the essential oils themselves; they have worked such miracles, taught me so many lessons, and have transformed so many lives.

Disclaimer

The information presented in this book is for educational purposes only. It is not intended in any way to be a substitute for professional medical care. Any application of the ideas, information, or techniques mentioned herein is undertaken at the reader's sole discretion and risk.

Much of the information about the actions of essential oils or the results of using them is based on the body of knowledge accumulated by the continuous use of certain plants throughout human history. This information is not necessarily based on scientific proof. It is in this spirit of traditional use that suggestions for the careful application of various oils are offered.

Table
of
Contents

Introduction

Aromatherapy may be defined as the therapeutic use of the essential oils of aromatic plants. These oils are highly concentrated forms of herbal energy, and represent the soul, or life force, of the plant. Extremely complex organic substances, they comprise hundreds of chemical compounds. Once extracted, they are quite volatile, and change from a highly potent liquid substance to an aromatic vapor in seconds when exposed to air. Their actions on the human body are not fully understood, but they have been used beneficially for thousands of years. At present, there are three main branches of aromatherapy:

1. Medical/clinical, an allopathic approach, in which most attention is paid to the chemical actions of the oils in enhancing the body's immune system and in attacking bacteria and viruses.

This approach originated in France, and is represented most notably by the work of the French physicians Valnet, Penoel, and Francômme.

2. Aesthetic, also referred to as aromacology, which concentrates on cosmetic applications.

3. Holistic, a "hands-on" therapy, employing massage and other body and energy therapies with the application of the essential oils. This approach is based on restoring the balance between body, mind, and spirit, employing the oils' psychological and emotional effects. It has been developed most fully in England, and is represented by the work of Madame Maury, Robert Tisserand, Patricia Davis, Shirley Price, and the author.

What do we really mean by holism? Plato once wrote:

> The cure of the part should not be attempted without the treatment of the whole. No attempts should be made to cure the body without the soul, and if the head and body are to be healthy you must begin by curing the mind, for this is the great error of our day in the treatment of the human body that physicians first separate the soul from the body.

A holistic perspective means looking at ourselves as an interpenetrating web of mind, body, and spirit, and also as a part of the larger environment in which we live. Our relationships with those around us, the values we live by, the society we are part of, our relationship to the planet we live on, even the way we are related to the rest of creation, all have bearing on what we manifest in our lives, right down to the simplest headache.

Meaning is an important element in holism, and it involves understanding connections between apparently unconnected elements. Is this headache just a headache (which it could be) or is it a symptom of something deeper (relationship problems, stress, a feeling of despair)? We may be carrying an emotional burden, feeling brokenhearted, or hungry for affection, and these feelings may manifest themselves physically.

they affect the physical body. The scent quality of the oils is unique in that the sense of smell can influence areas of the brain inaccessible to conscious control, such as emotions and hormonal responses. Application of the oils in massage can enhance the benefits of body work on the muscular, lymphatic, and nervous systems. By cutaneous application of the essential oils, we can influence more deeply the main body systems.

On the energetic level, aromatic oils are very active, and Margarite Maury conveyed this when she wrote, "…when we are dealing with an essential oil and its odoriferance we are dealing directly with a vital force, and entering the very heart of the alchemy of creation."

We will discuss the nature and properties of essential oils in subsequent chapters. What I want to convey here is that aromatherapy is a therapeutic system that has influences far beyond those immediately apparent, because of the special nature of the substances we are using.

Health is based on completeness and harmony in all aspects of life, and any therapy we employ should address this. There is no use treating a physical symptom if the underlying factors are not recognized. Aromatherapy can begin to approach some of these factors. We can use essential oils to help relieve various states of mind such as depression, to help bring our emotions into focus, to work on some of the physical manifestations of imbalance, and indeed to help us gain deeper knowledge about ourselves by using them in meditation.

This is why the essential oils have such an important role in a holistic approach: they work on so many levels. On a broader scale, they are products of our natural environment, and we are using remedies that are supportive of our natural life force which continually tries to maintain homeostasis.

In using essential oils in this way, we should look very carefully at all aspects of a client's life, and create a blend of oils appropriate to the individual's mental, emotional, spiritual, and physical situation. This is the basis of all true aromatherapy treatment, and is what Madame Maury was aiming at when she invented her Individual Prescription. The goal of this book is to present this approach to aromatherapy.

Origins of Aromatherapy

No one knows when mankind began using aromatic plants for healing purposes. We are reasonably sure that ancient man's senses were far more acute, and his sense of smell was crucial to his survival. There is evidence from the Neolithic period that aromatic herbs were used in cooking and medicine, and that herbs and flowers were buried with the dead. Smoking or fumigation was likely one of the earliest uses of plants, as part of ritual offerings to the gods. It was probably noticed that the smoke of various aromatic plants had hallucinogenic, stimulating, calming, or other effects. Gradually, a body of knowledge about plants accumulated and passed down the hundreds of generations of shamans.

Ancient Egypt was one of the civilizations where the use of aromatic medicine became highly developed. Of course, by that time China and India had advanced concepts of medicine, and you may wish to investigate the Eastern traditions in the use of aromatics. I will concentrate on the historical development most relevant to the Western herbal traditions.

The ritual use of aromatics was important in Egyptian spiritual life. Initially, priests and priestesses were the only people who had access to these precious substances. The earliest Egyptian use of aromatics was in incense, and it was thought that the smoke would rise to the abode of the gods. Frankincense was offered to the sun god Ra at sunrise, and myrrh belonged to the moon. The word "perfume" derives from the Latin *per* (through) and *fumum* (smoke, steam, vapor). In other words, "incense." One of the most famous Egyptian aromatic formulas was a mixture of 16 aromatic substances. It was known as *kyphi* and was made originally as a solid incense. Eventually it became a common item in Egyptian homes, and later was used as a liquid perfume by the Romans and Greeks.

No discussion of ancient Egyptian practice would be complete without mentioning the use of aromatics in mummification. Because the Egyptians believed that the dead would need the body in the afterlife, extreme measures were used to insure its preservation. The internal organs were removed and the cavity was filled with cassia and myrrh. The body was left to dehydrate for 70 days, and then wrapped in bandages impregnated with cedarwood oil and other aromatics. At the time of burial the body was decorated with flowers and a prayer was offered to the god Horus, requesting him to bestow his perfume on the body. The antiseptic qualities of the aromatics used in embalming helped to preserve the body.

The cedarwood used in embalming was most likely imported from Lebanon, and spikenard, myrrh, frankincense, labdanum, and cinnamon were imported from Babylon, Ethiopia, Somalia, Persia, and India. The Egyptians used these substances in unguents, perfumes, medicines, and cosmetics, and were known as expert perfumers all over the ancient world. An early Egyptian wrinkle cream contained the gums of frankincense and cypress, oils we still use today for aging skin. The Egyptians extracted oils using an infusion method, although some historians believe they had a primitive form of distillation.

The Papyrus Ebers, one of the few surviving medical papyri, describes the ingestion of aromatic medicines for internal problems, external application for pain, ointments for skin diseases, inhalations for respiratory ailments, gargles for mouth disorders, sitz baths and douches for gynecological disorders, and enemas for intestinal infections. Modern aromatherapists use the same methods.

When the Jews began their journey to the promised land about 1249 B.C., Moses was given instruction from Jehovah in the making of holy oil and incense:

> And the Lord said to Moses, "Take sweet spices, stacte, and onycha, and galbanum, sweet spices with pure frankincense (of each shall there be an equal part), and make an incense blended as by the perfumer, seasoned with salt, pure and holy;" … "And the incense which you shall make according to its composition, you shall not make for yourselves; it shall be for you holy to the Lord."[1]

There are many other references in the Bible to the use of aromatics for purification. Myrrh was used in the purification of Jewish women, and was worn around the neck as a deodorant and antiseptic while crossing the desert. Other references are found in The Song of Solomon, the birth of Christ, His anointment as King, and in His healing ministry. The continual link between aromatic substances and spirituality underlines the special nature of these plants.

The Greeks learned a great deal from the Egyptians about the use of aromatics. The invention of perfumes was attributed to the gods; men gained knowledge of them from the nymph Aeone. Aesculapius and Aphrodite were gods of healing, and healing essences and treatments were given by the priestesses in the temple of Aphrodite.

More importantly, Greek physicians began recording and classifying the properties of medicinal plants. Marestheus recognized that aromatic plants had stimulating or sedative qualities. Rose and hyacinth were considered refreshing and invigorating, lily and narcissus were sedative and hypnotic.

Long discussions took place over where on the body to apply the unguents. Diogenes felt the feet were best, as the scent would rise as the unguent melted. Anacreon thought the breast was best, because it was the seat of the heart and soul. Some wealthy Greeks anointed different parts of the body with different scents. The Greeks recognized that oils applied externally can affect internal organs and tissues. Hippocrates wrote that aromatic baths were useful in treating female disorders. Asclepiades believed that treatment should be pleasurable and recommended massage, music, perfume, bathing, and wine.

Discorides, the famous Greek physician, wrote a five-volume treatise on herbal medicine, describing the plants of the Mediterranean region. One of the sections dealt with aromatics, and the properties he ascribed to these plants have been verified throughout history. For example, myrrh strengthens gums, juniper is a diuretic, marjoram is soporific, and cypress stops bleeding. He could have been writing a modern book on aromatherapy.

The name Cleopatra is synonymous with beauty, seduction, and perfume; although more Greek than Egyptian, she was the last of the Egyptian queens. The art of manufacturing cosmetics and perfumes was well developed by her time, and she used the secrets of perfume in her seduction of Mark Antony.

The Romans were well-known for their spas and bath houses, and aromatics were used extensively in their daily lives. By this time, the common people had access to them. Entire sections of the city were occupied by the *unguentarii,* or perfumers. They had different names for three different types of perfume: *ladysmata* were the solid unguents, *stymmata* were scented oils, and *diapasmata* were powdered perfumes. They used aromatics to perfume hair, bodies, clothes, beds, flags, even walls of houses. A famous Roman oil was *nardinium,* which included calamus, costus, cardamom, melissa, spikenard, and myrrh.

Galen was a Greek who served as Royal Physician to the Roman Emperor and his family. He was also known for his work as surgeon at the School of Gladiators. It was said that his healing ability was so great that no gladiator ever died of wounds while he was responsible for their care. Galen's extensive knowledge of plant remedies was evident in his writings, and he classified plants into categories which are still known as Galenic.

"Lavender" comes from the Latin word *lavare* (to wash), perhaps stemming from its use in cleansing wounds. It's thought the Romans brought lavender to northern Europe during their occupation.

After the fall of Rome, many of the surviving physicians fled to Constantinople, where they became familiar with the Arabic understanding of aromatics. One of the most significant developments in the history of perfumery and aromatics was the perfection of distillation by Avicenna in the tenth century, although some historians believe that the Egyptians had a primitive form of distillation centuries before.

Rose was the first oil Avicenna distilled. Perfume as we know it, without a heavy oil base, now became possible. Rose water became an exportable commodity in the Arab world.

Middle Eastern aromatics and perfumes were brought to Europe by the Crusaders, and this stimulated the creation of the French perfume industry. French perfumers were granted their first charter in 1190 A.D. This led to the cultivation of aromatic plants for the perfumery trade in Europe, and made perfume more available for the gentry. The perfumers had little idea of the medicinal properties of the essential oils they were extracting.

In the twelfth century, Latin translations of the classic Greek writers such as Dioscorides began appearing in Europe, and in the fourteenth century an herbal revival began, perhaps prompted by the onset of the Black Death (bubonic plague). English manuscripts of the fourteenth and fifteenth centuries referred to infused oils, and gave instructions for making them. They discussed applying them externally, at the front and back of the body, for internal disorders. *Bancke's Herbal,* the first printed herbal, published in 1527, gives recipes for making an infused rose oil and instructions for its use:

> Oil of roses is made thus. Some boil roses in oil and keep it. Some do fill a vessel of glass with roses and oil, and they boil it in a cauldron full of water, and this oil is good. Some stamp fresh roses with oil, and they put it in a vessel of glass and set in the sun fifty days, and this oil is good against the chafing of the liver, if it be anointed therewith.

The perfection of distillation was linked to alchemy, and in sixteenth-century Germany several books appeared which dealt with distillation and essential oils. Among the alchemical writers was Hieronymus Braunschweig. In his last book written in 1597, he referred to 25 essential oils, including rosemary, lavender, clove, cinnamon, myrrh, and nutmeg. Much of what was written referred to alchemical processes, and the making of essential oils was an outcome of the search for the quintessence or spirit of the plant. The repeated distillation of the material, which also symbolized spiritual purification, led to the creation of potent medicinal substances.

Herbalists of this time were influenced by alchemical ideas, as well as Greek ideas on humors and plant energetics. Remedies were described as hot, cold, dry, and moist. The idea of the four elements (Air, Water, Fire, and Earth) and their corresponding humors formed the basis for prescribing. The humors were: Sanguine, Phlegmatic, Choleric, and Melancholic. Any imbalance could cause disease. The physician's job was to restore equilibrium by his choice of remedy. Thus we see that, along with astrological considerations and the doctrine of signatures, the medicine of this period was based on ancient ideas of the nature of the universe.

The return of the bubonic plague in the seventeenth century greatly increased the demand for aromatics, for they were the only known antiseptics. It was rumored that the perfumers and glove makers were relatively immune (there was a fashion for perfumed gloves at the time). Pomanders containing aromatic plants were worn or carried to ward off the disease.

It was believed that the plague was carried in the air, and large-scale fumigations were performed. Fires were lit in the city streets every 12 hours, and aromatic woods such as pine were burned. Incense and scented candles were burned indoors and in sick rooms, and floors were strewn with herbs. Culpeper[2] gives the following recipe:

A Pomander for the Time of Pestilence
Take of labdanum, styrax-calmite each one dram, cloves
half a dram, camphure, nard, nutmeg, each seven granes,

bruise them all to a fine powder, and mix them with rose water in which tragacanth and gum-arabick have been steeped, and make balls.

By the eighteenth century, aromatics were widely used by herbalists and some physicians. The earlier invention of printing had given the literate public access to herbal knowledge. Apothecaries supplied the essential oils and had shops where the public could buy remedies. The profession of medicine and the beginnings of chemistry began to develop at this time, and gradually a split appeared between the use of herbs and chemical drugs. Research into the active constituents of medicinal plants began, and the more mystical ideas like humors started to lose favor. Essential oils were still used extensively, and remained in the pharmacopoeia for some time. The developing power struggle between the rising profession of physician and the traditional herbalists has led some historians to suggest that the witch burnings may have been a way of eliminating competition by the village wise woman.

In the nineteenth century, the active principles of essences were investigated more scientifically than had been possible before, and in Witla's *Materica Medica* of 1882, 22 officially accepted essences were mentioned. The French researchers Cadeac and Meunier, and the Italians Gatti and Cajola published works on essential oils about this time. In 1887 Chamberland published his findings on the antiseptic powers of the vapors of essential oils, and also reported that the microorganisms of glanders and yellow fever were killed by them. Cinnamon, thyme, lavender, sandalwood, and cedarwood were found to be most powerful antibacterials. Even though essential oils were known to be effective, synthesized chemical medicines were becoming increasingly popular.

It was not until the early 1930s that the therapeutic use of essential oils was finally given a name, "Aromatherapie," and considered to be a discipline in its own right. A chemist in the family perfumery business, Rene-Maurice Gattefosse spent 50 years researching essential oils, fragrance, and the therapeutic and psychological effect of aromas, and was aware that he was laying the foundation for further work in the field. His famous work, *Aromatherapie,* published in 1937, was an important landmark in aromatherapy literature, although Monsieur Gattefosse had previously authored a number of works on perfumery early on in the century. In the 1920s he wrote about the therapeutic properties of essential oils in *Reflections on the Use of Essential Oils, Physiological Role of Perfumes, Physiological Action of Aromatic Solutions,* and *Therapeutic Uses of Bergamot Oil.* He also published several books on the use of aromatherapy in dermatology and esthetics in the 1940s. Having devoted a lifetime to understanding essential oils and their therapeutic effects, Rene-Maurice Gattefosse must be regarded as one of the main figures in modern aromatherapy.

In an article written in 1936, Gattefosse described Aromatherapie (the name he invented) as: "…a therapy employing aromatics in a sphere of research opening enormous vistas to those who have started exploring it."

Other people were exploring the possibilities of essential oils at that time. In Los Angeles a Mr. Godissant was using essential oils for treating skin cancer, gangrene, and other skin problems. Roland Hunt wrote a book about aromatherapy during this period. In Australia, Penfold was researching tea-tree oil, and in Italy the psychotherapeutic actions of essential oils were being investigated.

World War II halted much of this activity. An exception was Dr. Valnet, a French army surgeon who experimented with essential oils for treating war wounds. He continued his research after the war, and his book[3] was published in 1964. Dr. Valnet introduced aromatherapy to the French medical profession, and it is now an accepted part of the French medical system.

Marguerite Maury was another notable figure in modern aromatherapy. She was a French biochemist who was uneasy about using the oils internally, and was also interested in rejuvenation. She did extensive research into the ancient use of aromatics, and devised a system of aromatherapy which used the oils externally in a system of massage, having become convinced that cutaneous absorption was the best method of introducing oils into the body. She also pioneered the idea of the Individual Prescription, which was a therapeutic blend absolutely unique for each client. Madame Maury went to England in the 1950s, and was principally responsible for the non-medical aromatherapy which developed there.

Madeline Arcier has carried on Madame Maury's work, and operates a clinic and school in London. Robert Tisserand's book,[4] Patricia Davis' London School of Aromatherapy and her books,[5] and Shirley Price's work and books[6] have done much to introduce holistic aromatherapy to the general public and gain its acceptance in British hospitals.

Endnotes

1. Holy Bible, Exodus 30, Verse 22.

2. Culpeper, N. *Culpeper's Complete Herbal.* London: W. Foulsham & Co.

3. Valnet, J. *The Practice of Aromatherapy.* Saffron Walden, England: C. W. Daniel, 1980.

4. Tisserand, R. *The Art of Aromatherapy.* Saffron Walden, England: C. W. Daniel, 1977.

5. Davis, P. *Aromatherapy: An A–Z.* Saffron Walden, England: C. W. Daniel, 1988.
   ————. *Subtle Aromatherapy.* Saffron Walden, England: C. W. Daniel, 1991.

6. Price, S. *Practical Aromatherapy: How to Use Essential Oils to Restore Vitality.* Wellingborough, England: Thorsons, 1983.
   ————. *Aromatherapy for Common Ailments.* London: Gaia Books Ltd., 1991.

2

The Life Force of the Plant

The *American Aromatherapy Association* defines essential oils as:

> ...highly concentrated, volatile extracts distilled from aromatic herbs, flowers, and trees, containing hormone-like properties, and natural antiseptics.

They have also been called the life force of the plant. According to Drs. Francômme and Penoel:

> Plant essences, in the physiological meaning of the term, are most certainly true life essences, elaborated by the secretory cells of the plants which have tapped the photo-electro-magnetic energy of the sun and have converted it, with the intervention of enzymes, into biochemical energy under the form of highly diversified aromatic molecules.[1]

Just because something is natural doesn't mean it is harmless. Essential oils are highly concentrated forms of plant energy. This is a very important property. **Your safety in using the oils, and the safety of those to whom you introduce them, depends on your understanding of this.** One drop of rose oil contains the energy from 30 roses, and one drop of essential oil is said to have the therapeutic value of 25 cups of herbal infusion. Two women have died trying to induce abortion with pennyroyal, and only 15 milliliters of wintergreen taken orally can be fatal.

Different plants produce different quantities of essential oil, and this determines the prices of essences. The amount obtainable varies from 0.01 to 10 percent. Rose contains very little essence, and up to 2,000 pounds of rose petals are needed to produce one pound of essential oil. On the other hand, to produce one pound of oil requires only 50 pounds of eucalyptus plant material, or 150 pounds of lavender, or 500 pounds of sage, thyme, or rosemary.

The volatility of essential oils is one of the things that distinguishes them from plant-based herbal remedies. It is the odoriferous molecules of essential oil which make up the "aroma" in aromatherapy, and which we inhale. Because of the different sizes, weights, and chemical composition of their molecules, essential oils have different evaporation rates and therapeutic effects on the body.

Perfumery terms for evaporation rates are top notes, middle notes, and base notes. These varying rates are measured numerically on the Poucher scale. Top notes evaporate quickly, and provide the initial impact in a blend. They are generally uplifting and stimulating. Top notes come from the citrus family, some herbs, and trees such as eucalyptus.

Middle notes form the substance of a blend, and seem to function on the metabolism of the body. They generally come from spices and herbs such as cinnamon and lavender.

The base notes bring solidity, fixity, and sedation. They act on the mucous membranes and are good for elderly people and people with chronic conditions. They generally are used in perfumery to fix or hold a blend, and come from woods, roots, and resins. Sandalwood, vetivert, and myrrh are good examples of base notes.

In addition to being extremely volatile, essences are affected by heat and light, and should be kept in dark glass bottles away from direct light and extremes of temperature. Some are very inflammable. It is important to know that many plastics are unsuitable for bottling because they are dissolved by essential oils.

Although essence oils are called oils, they are not really oily substances, but have a viscosity more like water. They are generally transparent, and can be various colors, such as blue (camomile), green (bergamot), and orange (tangerine). They are soluble in alcohol, oil, or fat, but not in water. The shelf life of essential oils (apart from citrus oils) if undiluted is generally up to six years or longer if stored correctly. Absolutes and resins have a much shorter shelf life.

Essential oils are usually secreted by special glands, ducts, or cells in different parts of plants, and are found in the sap and wood of certain trees. They can be found in roots, stems, bark, leaves, fruits and flowers, and are more abundant in some botanical families than others. The plant families which seem to be most prolific in essential oil production are: *Lamiaceae, Myrtacae, Cupressaceae, Rutacea, Lauraceae,* and *Apiaceae.*

Following is a list of essential oils and the parts of plants from which they are derived.

Roots: ginger, vetivert, angelica.

Leaves and stems: basil, cajeput, clary sage, cypress, eucalyptus, geranium, hyssop, marjoram, myrtle, lemon, verbena, melissa, niaouli, oregano, petitgrain, patchouli, pine needle, peppermint, rosemary, sage, savory, spearmint, spruce, tea-tree, thyme, tarragon.

Bark: cinnamon, birch.

Flowers: camomile, jasmine, neroli, rose, ylang-ylang, calendula, lavender.

Flower buds: clove.

Fruit peels: grapefruit, bergamot, mandarin, orange, lemon, lime, tangerine.

Seeds: carrot, fennel, caraway, coriander, aniseed, nutmeg.

Resins: frankincense, benzoin, myrrh, galbanum, elemi.

Wood: sandalwood, camphor, cedarwood, rosewood.

Grasses: citronella, lemongrass, palmarosa.

Essences from different parts of the same plant can have different chemical structures, as in cinnamon bark and leaves. The same plant can also secrete quite different essential oils. For example, both petit-grain and neroli come from the bitter orange tree.

Climate has much to do with the quantity and quality of essential oil produced. Most of our essential oils come from areas of the world with hot climates: the Mediterranean region, the Middle East, India, Australia, and the Pacific Islands. The chemical composition of the essential oil varies with the time of year, the time of day, the condition of the soil, the variety of plant, etc. The best time to harvest jasmine is at sunset when the essence is at its highest level in the flower. Ylang-ylang is harvested in May or June, because that is when its flowers yield the highest percentage of oil.

Plants rely on light for their biochemical processes, and the type of light they receive affects the therapeutic action of the essential oil. At sea level, sunlight reaching the plant has traveled through the entire atmosphere. Because of scattering and absorption by air molecules, dust, smoke, etc., the spectrum of the light may be weak in the blue and violet wavelengths. A plant growing in this environment will produce more phenol. At high altitudes, the thinner atmosphere produces less scattering and consequently less loss of these wavelengths. The same plant growing in the mountains will produce more alcohols. Botanically, they are the same plant, but they are very different therapeutically.

Classic Methods of Production

Traditionally, essential oils have been produced in four main ways: distillation, enfleurage, cold expression, and solvent extraction. Steam distillation is the method used to produce most essential oils.

In this method, the plant material is placed on a wire mesh in a large copper or stainless steel vat. Steam is passed through the plant material, the heat causes the odoriferous glands to rupture, and the essence is released in the form of vapor.

The vaporous mixture of water and essence is collected in a special tube called a "swan neck" and sent to a refrigerated coil, where the vapor is condensed. The water and essential oil separate naturally upon cooling because of their different specific gravities, the essential oil usually being lighter than water. As the essence separates, it runs into a collecting vessel known as a Florentine flask.

The liquid left over, called a hydrolate or distillate, contains the water-soluble components of the plants distilled. It may be floral or herbal water, and can be used in skin care, with children, or whenever a milder effect is desired.

On some large farms, the plants are distilled as soon as they are harvested, because the essential oil is a very delicate substance. Examples of distilled essential oils are: lavender, basil, clove, cypress, eucalyptus, geranium, marjoram, rosemary, nutmeg, peppermint, sage, sandalwood, thyme, and ylang-ylang.

Enfleurage, one of the oldest methods of extracting the essences, is based on the fact that the essential oils dissolve in fat. In this method, purified fat or wax is spread over glass trays and the plants are placed on top of the fat. Every day the flowers or plants are changed, until the fat or wax is saturated with essential oil. A solvent such as alcohol is then used to separate out the essence. This is an old Egyptian method, and was used to extract the essences from delicate flowers such as rose and jasmine. Sometimes the process takes as long as seven weeks. Oils produced by this method are called concretes, and are very concentrated. These concretes are further processed to yield absolutes. This method is so costly and time-consuming that it has largely been replaced by the use of chemical solvents.

In the solvent extraction method, the flowers or plants are immersed in a suitable solvent such as acetone, alcohol, ether, or benzine. The mixture is heated until the solvent has evaporated, leaving the essential oil in the container. Flower absolutes such as rose, jasmine, and neroli are often produced this way, since they are too delicate for distillation, and also have small concentrations of essential oil in the flowers. The absolutes produced by this method should not be taken internally, because they may still contain traces of the chemicals used.

Cold expression is the method which produces the most natural essential oil, because no heat or chemical treatment is involved. This is the method most frequently used to extract citrus oils. Originally, rinds of the citrus fruit were squeezed by hand until the little essential oil globules burst. The oil was collected in a sponge, which was then squeezed into a container. Now this process is usually done mechanically.

The Purity of Essential Oils

The therapeutic efficacy of an essential oil will depend on its purity. Many studies have shown that the whole essential oil operates synergistically, and is always more effective than the sum of its parts, or just its major chemical constituent. It is important to work with high quality, pure essential oils whenever you can. Many of the oils on the market are of poor quality.

The major consumers of essential oils are the perfume and food industries. Robert Tisserand says that aromatherapists use only about two percent of the essential oil supply, with the food-flavoring industry using 50 percent, the pharmaceutical industry 20 percent, and the fragrance industry 25 percent. (Since this was written, essential oils used in aromatherapy have become much more important as a factor in total oil consumption.)

Absolute purity in these fields is not as important as in aromatherapy; in fact, the perfume industry has been moving away from natural essences for some time. Most perfumes contain only a small percentage of essential oils, and the perfume industry requires a much larger range of scents than pure essential oils can provide.

If an essential oil is to be suitable for aromatherapy, it should be from the correct plant source, harvested at the right time, and grown under the correct conditions, preferably organically. It should never be adulterated with chemicals or synthetics.

What to Look for in Essential Oils

- The oil should smell like the plant it comes from. This is a simple guide, but one that many people ignore. When you inhale the oil you should feel its effect in your body, unlike synthetic oils, which will feel irritating.

- Oils should be clear, not cloudy, and straw colored, or green, brown, orange, etc. They should not be greasy and should evaporate cleanly.

- They should be priced differently. Do not buy uniformly-priced essences. Rose oil should be far more expensive than rosemary. If it is not, it may be diluted, synthetic, or extended. Low prices may also mean the oil is a second or third distillation of the plant material, in which case it will have far less therapeutic value. Sometimes oils are diluted with another plant that has a similar aroma, but costs less; for example, citronella is often sold as melissa. Real melissa oil is actually more expensive than rose. Obtaining the specific oil you want is more likely if you know the correct botanical name of the plant, provided that the supplier is truthful. "Marigold" can be either calendula or tagetes. Since there is no essential oil of marigold produced, calendula or marigold oil is always a macerated oil (vegetable oil in which the flowers have been soaked).

- The oils should be sold in dark glass bottles, definitely not in plastic.

- The part of the plant the oil comes from is important. For example, cinnamon bark oil and cinnamon leaf oil are very irritating to the skin. Juniper berry oil is far superior to oil distilled from juniper leaves.

Common Methods of Adulteration

- A certain quantity of the main chemical constituent may be added to the essential oil to "stretch" it.

- Oil from a cheaper plant may be added. Citronella may be added to melissa; spearmint is often added to birch.

- Synthetic aromatic substances may be added. This can cause irritation, allergies, nausea, headaches, and reduced therapeutic value.

- Some of the chemical constituents may be removed. Since an essential oil is an extremely complex cocktail of hundreds of chemical constituents, some of them in very small amounts, this will alter the therapeutic value of the oil. Menthol is often removed from peppermint oil and used by the pharmaceutical industry. As a general rule, the more an essential oil is interfered with physically or chemically, the less clinical value it will have.

The Role of Essential Oils in the Plant

The complete role of essences in the life of plants is not fully understood. I will describe some functions, but much research remains to be done on the full significance of these marvelous substances.

In plants which produce flower oils, one of the obvious functions is to attract insects for pollination, which insures reproduction and survival of the species. Red and pink flowers, about nine percent of the aromatic flowers, attract butterflies by both color and scent. White flowers, which attract moths, account for about 15 percent of aromatic blooms. Morris[2] says that the night-blooming flowers are white because they reflect the moonlight better than other colors and this helps guide the moth to the flower. This type of flower also has a heavy, languorous, sweet scent which attracts the moth. Jasmine, lilies, hyacinths, and honeysuckle are examples of this type of flower.

A Chinese emperor moth can detect a scent six miles downwind. Bees are attracted to yellow, lavender, and blue flowers and the scents associated with them.

Another basic function of essences in the plant is to protect it against predators. Within the plant, the essences are separated from the plant tissues because they can be toxic to them. Pine oil, for example, damages plant tissue even at a dilution of 1 to 50,000 parts.

The strength of the oil keeps away predators because it can burn the mouth of an animal attempting to eat the plant. In the Mediterranean region, goats known to eat almost anything will not touch the pungent herbs such as wild thyme and wild marjoram. Sandalwood is impervious to termites; cedar and redwood trees are also highly resistant to various insect pests.

Another way that essences protect their plants is to reduce dehydration. Evaporation of oils from the leaves appears to inhibit the transpiration of water vapor. Interestingly, the plants containing the highest percentage of essential oils are generally found in the warm, sunny parts of the world. An environmental adaptation, perhaps?

The Chemistry of Essential Oils

The chemical composition of an essential oil is what produces its particular aroma and its biological effects. Although chemists have isolated and identified many of the complex compounds found in essences, Valnet[3] notes that essential oils present researchers with more new compounds than all the chemists in the world could analyze in a thousand years. Valnet also says:

> The whole natural essence is found to be more active than its principal constituent. Moreover, those constituents which form a smaller percentage of the whole are found to be more active than those of its principal constituent. As early as 1904 Cuthbert Hall demonstrated that the antiseptic properties of the essence of eucalyptus were more powerful than those of its principal constituent, eucalyptol.

This is an important point, for it means that the synthesis of an oil by using its main constituents, or extracting one main constituent, can never produce results as effective as those obtained by using the entire natural oil. Some plants produce oils which contain a compound that can cause undesirable side effects, but other substances in the essence offset them.

Hoffman[4] cites salicylic acid. This compound, commonly known as aspirin, is found in wintergreen and birch oils. Used alone, it can cause stomach hemorrhage, but some plants containing it along with other compounds can actually stop stomach bleeding. Hoffman notes that the herb meadowsweet has this property.

The main chemical constituents and their principal modes of action are listed below, with examples of oils which contain high percentages of the compound.

Acids: These are principally antiseptics. Wintergreen contains salicyclic acid, and benzoin has a high benzoic acid content.

Alcohols: Linalol and terpinol are common. They are germicides with low toxicity, which is important in long-term use. Oils with high alcohol content are frequently used in skin care preparations. They are energizing, toning, deodorizing, and antiseptic, and have some of the most pleasing, fruity aromas. Examples are bergamot, lavender, and geranium.

Aldehydes: These tend to be calming and anti-inflammatory. They are found in abundance in the grasses. Examples are lemon balm (melissa), lemon verbena, and lemongrass.

Cetones or Ketones: Cetones ease the secretion of mucus and also help stimulate the growth of new skin cells. They can be toxic, so care should be taken in long-term use. Two cetones commonly found in oils are carvone (dill) and verbenon (rosemary). Eucalyptus, hyssop, and rosemary all have high cetone content.

Esters: These are soothing, calming, and fungicidal. They are electrically neutral, balancing, and tend to a greenish color. Lavender has a high ester content, as do benzoin, geranium, and neroli.

Phenols: Phenols have the strongest antiseptic qualities found in essential oils. They are irritating, hot, and very stimulating. Long-term use can produce some liver toxicity. Eugenol, thymol, and carvacrol are phenols commonly found in oils. Clove, oregano, and thyme have high phenol content.

Terpenes: These tend to be antibiotic in nature. They are stimulants and skin irritants, and are reputed to be effective antiseptics in vapor form against *Meningococcus, Staphylococcus,* and *Typhus bacillus.* Valnet cites research showing that lemon and thyme oils appear to be the most effective. Pine contains a high percentage of the terpene pinene.

Oils which have been classified very precisely according to their unique chemical profiles are called chemotypes. Different species of the same plant genus, or even plants of the same species grown in different environments, can have quite different chemical compositions, and chemotyping enables the therapist to choose exactly the treatment effect wanted.

Thyme, rosemary, tea-tree, and eucalyptus oils have been extensively chemotyped. *Eucalyptus radiata* has few cetonic compounds; on the other hand, *Eucalyptus globulus* has more cetones, so is more toxic and must be diluted more than other eucalyptus chemotypes. Thyme can be thyme with thymol, or thyme with linalol, the latter being more gentle. The three chemotypes of rosemary act on different parts of the body. The borneol type is a good general stimulant, the cineole type is a good pulmonary antiseptic, and the verbenon type is more specific to the liver and gall bladder. All of them share the general characteristics of rosemary. See the Appendix for detailed information about 24 essential oils.

Endnotes

1. Francômme, P. *Phytoguide No. 1: Aromatherapy, Advanced Therapy for Infectious Illnesses.* La Courtete, France: International Phytomedical Foundation, 1985.

2. Morris, E. *Fragrance.* Greenwich: E. T. Morris & Co., 1984.

3. Valnet, J. *The Practice of Aromatherapy.* Saffron Walden, England: C. W. Daniel, 1980.

4. Hoffman, D. *The Holistic Herbal.* Forris, Scotland: The Findham Press, 1983.

3

The Aromatic Symphony

Blending oils is one of the most exciting and creative activities in aromatherapy. It is also one of the most important, because making individual therapeutic blends is the basis of your work as an aromatherapist. Once you have a thorough knowledge of the oils, blending will begin to come naturally, but you also need to have some knowledge of the two principal types of blending, aesthetic and therapeutic.

Aesthetic Blending

Perfumery is the ancient art of blending scents to produce a particular scent quality. It involves understanding the different types of scents, how they work together, and the ability to produce a perfume that is more than the sum of its parts. Scent quality is important in aromatherapy because it is necessary to produce a blend that is pleasing to the person using it. Little benefit can be obtained from something that offends the nose! We also know that aromatic substances can have strong psychological effects. They can be relaxing, uplifting, refreshing, antidepressant, arousing, and so forth. The whole perfume industry is based on this. Perfumers have developed an entire vocabulary to describe scents and their qualities. We can use these ideas to help our understanding and increase our appreciation of this elusive and magical realm.

The main categories for classifying scents in perfumery and the corresponding essential oils are listed below.

Florals: Jasmine, neroli, rose, camomile (not used in perfumery), lavender, and ylang-ylang.

Green notes: These are created to reproduce the scent of a crushed green leaf. Pine, mint, marjoram, rosemary, basil, and other herbal oils are used. Sometimes lavender is used as a bridge between the florals and the green notes.

Citrus: Lemon, orange, tangerine, grapefruit, and bergamot. Neroli is sometimes used, and petitgrain.

Oriental: These are the heavy, heady perfumes and include spices (cinnamon and clove), resins (frankincense), and woods (sandalwood and cedarwood).

Chrypre: These are soft, warm, and sweet-smelling perfumes, and include such things as gum labdanum, oakmoss, and bergamot.

Aldehydic: Very popular in modern perfumery. They have a lot of top notes and are energetic. Examples are lemongrass and melissa.

Leather/animal scents: These are not used in aromatherapy, in perfumery they are represented by civet, musk, ambergris, and birch tar.

"Tenacity" is the ability of a fragrance to last a long time. Fixatives with high molecular weight are used to prolong the tenacity of a fragrance. In aromatherapy we would use a heavy essential oil such as sandalwood, patchouli, or myrrh to fix a blend.

The body of a perfume means the balance among the top notes, middle notes, and base notes. A perfume that is not well-balanced will be perceived as "thin," so a balanced blend is important. In blending a commercial perfume, it is desirable to create a symphony of scent, which has many tones and layers that unfold in an interesting way in time. When wearing perfume, you probably have noticed that the scent is quite different two hours after its application. You will smell the top notes first, then the middle and the base notes, although a good perfume will be more subtle and there may be layers upon layers. Also, the perfume interacts with your body chemistry and hence will smell different on different people.

Creating a great perfume is much like creating a work of art. Scents are used as a painter uses his colors, and inspiration can come from many sources. It has been said that Henri Robert, a master perfumer for the house of Chanel, kept a diary of fragrance perceptions that he had observed during his worldwide travels.

The devotion of the master perfumers to their art leads them to work with equally excellent designers to create exactly the right packages for their creations, and names are chosen, almost like a mantra, to encapsulate the spirit of the perfume. This emphasizes the point that certain smells can create realities for us that we would not necessarily enter in any other way.

The great noses of the world can detect any of the thousands of synthetic and natural ingredients now used in perfumes, which shows that the sense of smell can be significantly improved by training and use. You will find as you work with the essential oils that you will become increasingly sensitive to your environment, not only in the olfactory sense, but also visually, tactually, and aesthetically. I believe that this happens because these substances are so pure and have such ethereal qualities.

One consequence of this is that when walking down the street, one becomes aware of the scents and living habits of all who pass by: the person who had garlic for breakfast, the one who hasn't bathed for days, the many cigarettes another person smoked last night, or the perfume on that perfectly respectable businessman's collar. It can make a simple shopping expedition quite a traumatic experience!

A note of caution is in order here. Many of the scents used in perfumery are synthetics. For example, anything sold as essential oil of honeysuckle, lily of the valley, carnation, or jonquil is very likely synthetic, because the oil yield from these plants is so low that the pure oil would be prohibitively expensive. The purity of the essence is not so important in perfumery, as long as the scent is what the designer wants. I must emphasize that such synthetics have no therapeutic value and no place in aromatherapy.

Following is a list of some of the classic perfumes in each of the major categories:

Floral: Joy by Paton, 1935.

Green: Chanel #19 by Chanel, 1971.

Aldehydes: Arpege by Lanvin, 1927.

Chypre: Miss Dior by Dior, 1947.

Oriental: Opium by Yves St. Laurent, 1952.

The following are some of the great men's perfumes:

Leather: Cuir de Russie by Chanel, 1924.

Fougere: Brut by Faberge, 1964.

Oriental: Old Spice.

Therapeutic Blending

We know that when we blend essential oils they form a molecular compound that cannot be separated again. Thus by blending we are creating an entirely new substance whose properties are more than the sum of its parts.

Although we are blending for therapeutic purposes, it's a good idea to use some of the laws of perfumery to create a balanced blend. Also we should try to ensure that the oils we are using will blend and work together harmoniously.

Some essential oils have a very strong odor, for example, eucalyptus and peppermint, so we may decide to use less of these to make the blend more acceptable to a client's nose. Lavender is one of the least intense oils, and we often add it to a blend to hold it together, or to tone down dominant oils.

Another consideration in blending is that some oils may be one-sided; that is, they may be very sweet or sour. Ylang-ylang is sickeningly sweet to many people, so it is often blended with citrus oils to cut the sweetness. Bergamot blends well with it. Jasmine is another sweet-smelling oil. Lemon is very sour and some blenders add lavender to soften it. Personal preferences play a large part, but you can add a drop or two of another oil to make the blend more acceptable, apart from the therapeutic factors.

Blending by plant family is a good way to create harmonious blends. You can blend flowers, or trees, citrus, or woods together and know that they will not clash. Examples of flower blends would be jasmine and geranium, or lavender and neroli. Some blenders assign colors to the oils according to their subjective interpretations of their properties, and blending by color can be an interesting exercise. For example, you could call cinnamon reddish-brown and ylang-ylang orange, and this would be a nice blend. You could try complementary colors and opposite colors. The colors can give you a feeling about the qualities of a blend.

You could think of oils as one of the four elements Fire, Earth, Air, and Water. If you decided that a client needed to get in touch with his or her emotions and needed "grounding," you could make a blend of earth and water oils. Culpeper[1] assigned the planets as rulers of certain plants; these could be used as astrological blends. Meditating with the oils, and writing down your feelings about them, is a good way to learn about their energetic qualities.

Some writers classify the oils as yin or yang. Yin oils can be considered as sedative and yang oils as stimulating. These are fundamental classifications in aromatherapy, and a good place to start when thinking about the properties required in a particular blend.

Once you get a feeling for the oils, blending becomes a creative experience, and using different ways of classifying oils and blending them is a good way to learn the essence of each one and how they work together. Keeping a blending notebook is an excellent idea.

Note the ingredients, proportions, whether the odor was pleasing, the effects, whether you would use it again, what it was used for and the response, and so forth.

Remembering that the essential oils work on physical, emotional, and psychological levels, we must make our blends accordingly. A good blend will fit the client like a glove and work towards balancing the mind and body. M. Maury[2] wrote:

> It is strange to discover the similarity between the impression produced by the composition of the perfume, and that given by the living person. Almost invariably, the odor, and above all the fragrance of the I.P. express and almost depict the person feature by feature. Gay or sad, charmer or sour. The impression, the sensation suggested by the perfume, are exactly the same as those felt on contact with the person.

The "I.P." (Individual Prescription) refers to the fact that the true art in aromatherapy lies in creating the perfect therapeutic blend for each individual person. General blends, such as a relaxing/stress-relieving blend will work because of the properties of the essential oils used, but a blend that fits the personality and physiology of the person for which it was created will work much better.

A good example is a headache blend. There are many kinds of headaches, with different underlying causes. Let's say that Mrs. Smith has a stress headache. Why is she stressed? Is it her job? Is it because she is hard on herself and demands perfection? Or perhaps her husband has just died and she has to deal with the details of his burial as well as her grief. How does the headache manifest itself? Is it tension at the back of her neck? Is it migraine? Are digestive or liver problems associated with it? For each of these possibilities we would use a different essential oil; for the new widow we might add rose to help her deal with the basic cause of her stress, bereavement.

You may ask how one could create an appropriate blend for this woman. One way is to make three lists: important emotional, psychological, and physical considerations. From each list pick two or three of the most immediate issues, then match essential oils to each issue.

Emotional issues:

Grief	→	Rose
Anger	→	Rose
Panic	→	Neroli

Psychological issues:

Can't focus on tasks	→	Rosemary
Feels very ungrounded	→	Vetivert
Stays up nights worrying	→	Lavender

Physical issues:

Upset digestive system	→	Camomile
Headaches	→	Lavender
Feels cold all the time	→	Ginger

Although other oils could be used for each issue, the ones shown illustrate the process. So we have a blend of rose, neroli, rosemary, vetivert, lavender, camomile, and ginger.

It's best not to put more than three or four oils in a blend, so I would make two blends for Mrs. Smith. Into the first, a grounding, stimulating blend, I would put rosemary, vetivert, and ginger. This would be good to use in the morning to help her think straight and deal with the practical problems she faces. The second blend, with rose, camomile, neroli, and lavender would be used in the evening to help her deal with the emotions that arise in the lonely evenings without her husband, and to help her sleep.

Shirley Price[3] has a good set of tables which can be a great help in selecting appropriate oils for each problem. Personal consultation is absolutely necessary to determine the situation you are dealing with. Reflexology or another diagnostic method can be helpful in deciding which oils to use at the physical level. Naturally, you must change the blend as the client's situation changes.

You must always be aware of any contraindications in formulating blends, and be sure to ask the client to smell the blend before you use it for massage or offer it as a bath blend. If he or she doesn't like the odor, try to substitute another oil; there are usually several that you can use. However, if you cannot use a substitute, don't use the objectionable substance. Always trust the person's own inner voice.

I work as an aromatherapist/massage therapist in a local chiropractor's office. The chiropractic assistant has developed a game of smelling the blends made for each client, and has begun to associate different blends with individual clients according to the "feeling" of the blend.

Sometimes she thinks a particular blend smells awful, but the client loves it, precisely because it's just what he or she needs at that time. This shows how subjective blending is. Remember, you don't have to like the blends you create for others, as long as they like them. When it's needed, even garlic can smell better than roses!

To determine the proportion of each oil in the blend, order your list of symptoms by importance and adjust the amount of each oil accordingly, not forgetting the total number of drops appropriate to the type of treatment you are doing. For example, if you're making a three percent massage blend and are using one ounce of carrier oil, your total of essential oils is 18 drops. Thus Mrs. Smith's morning blend could have eight drops of rosemary, six of vetivert, and four of ginger. When using a hot oil like ginger, I wouldn't put more than three or four drops in a blend.

If all this seems pretty complicated at this point, don't despair. With experience and a love of the oils, you will develop a feeling for blending and will find an exciting adventure of discovery in creating and experimenting with new blends.

Endnotes

1. Culpeper, N. *Culpeper's Complete Herbal.* London: W. Foulsham & Co.

2. Maury, M. *Marguerite Maury's Guide to Aromatherapy: The Secret of Life and Youth.* Saffron Walden, England: C. W. Daniel, 1989.

3. Price, S. *Practical Aromatherapy: How to Use Essential Oils to Restore Vitality.* Wellingborough, England: Thorsons, 1987.

Applied Aromatics

Using essential oils correctly is one of the most important things to know if you are to get the full benefit of their properties. Choosing the correct method, knowing the correct dilutions, and being aware of the possible contraindications of specific oils will ensure that you are using them safely and responsibly. As mentioned earlier, the pure oils are highly concentrated, potent substances. Treat them with respect, and the magic they can perform will surprise you.

Baths

One of the most common methods of use is in the bath. This sounds simple, but indeed is a very effective method, because the oil can act in two ways: by penetration of the skin, and by inhalation, since the warm water causes evaporation and the creation of an aromatic cloud in the bathroom (provided that you close the door). We know that inhalation can effect mood changes, act on our respiratory system, and allow the oil to enter the bloodstream via the lungs.

Although the primary method of application in holistic aromatherapy is massage, baths can be an excellent way of using oils with someone who is reluctant to, or cannot be massaged. Water has always been used as a healing medium, and the combination of oils and water seems to create a third force. The warmth also is very comforting and relaxing. What could be more therapeutic than a perfumed bath? However, don't use bubble bath, synthetic scents, or soap in an aromatherapy bath, just essential oils.

Full baths, sitz baths, foot baths, and hand baths all can be effective. Foot baths can be used to treat colds, headaches, migraines, leg disorders, varicose veins, and menstrual problems. They are restorative after a long day on your feet, or in cases of extreme fatigue. The French herbalist, Maurice Messigue used foot and hand baths extensively in his treatments. They were his favorite methods and he believed they were so effective because the hands and feet are the most receptive parts of the body. This is not surprising if we remember that the body's meridians end there, and, according to reflexology, the hands and feet have reflex areas that relate to the entire body.

For a full bath, run the bath, turn off the water, and then add the essences. If you add them while the water is running, they will evaporate too quickly, and your ceiling will get the benefit! The standard dosage for a full bath is six to eight drops of essential oil. For a foot or hand bath, use two to three drops. With citrus oils such as lemon, spice oils such as cinnamon, and peppermint, use no more than three drops, because it is easy to "burn" the skin with these oils. If you do use too much and get burned, which feels like a prickly sensation, or if you get a rash, get out of the bath immediately and apply jojoba or some other vegetable oil. The vegetable oil will dilute the essential oil. Because the essential oils are not water-soluble, you can't wash them off with water.

A good example of a "burn" is the following experience we had with cinnamon oil. Although I'm usually very careful about leaving essential oils around the house, there is always a chance for a mistake. My husband got into the bathtub and accidentally knocked a bottle of cinnamon oil onto his lower back. The oil spilled directly on his skin and left an angry red burn mark about three inches long down his backside. This lasted for several months, and was a source of great embarrassment to me, the professional aromatherapist!

Messigue suggests taking foot baths in the morning with an empty stomach, if they are used as a treatment method. He believes that they should last no more than eight minutes. Hand baths should be taken in the evening before eating, and again should be limited to eight minutes. Both types of bath should be as hot as possible.

Here are some recipes for therapeutic baths:

A stimulating morning bath

peppermint 2 drops
rosemary 4 drops
juniper 2 drops

A calming evening bath

lavender 4 drops
marjoram 4 drops

A warming stimulating bath

ginger 2 drops
rosemary 4 drops
lavender 2 drops

A cooling summer bath

peppermint 2 drops
eucalyptus 4 drops
lemon 2 drops

A cleansing detoxifying bath

lemon 2 drops
juniper 4 drops
geranium 2 drops

An aphrodisiac bath
 vetivert 3 drops
 ylang-ylang 3 drops
 mandarin 2 drops

A muscular aches and pains bath
 marjoram 3 drops
 clary sage 3 drops
 rosemary 2 drops

A menstrual pain/PMS bath
 clary sage 4 drops
 peppermint 1 drop
 juniper 3 drops
(Can be used as a sitz bath with half amounts of drops.)

A foot bath for tired feet
 lavender 1 drop
 peppermint 1 drop
 cypress 1 drop

A foot bath for varicose veins
 cypress 2 drops
 lemon 1 drop

A sitz bath for cystitis
 bergamot 2 drops
 sandalwood 1 drop
 juniper 1 drop

Massage

Massage is the method of application of essential oils in holistic aromatherapy. We will discuss all the benefits of aromatherapy massage in Chapter 8, and will explain how the oils penetrate the skin and are absorbed into the blood stream and lymphatic system.

The type of massage used is generally a gentle, relaxing one, and utilizes the various energy systems of the body. The percussive techniques of Swedish massage or deep tissue work are not suitable for aromatherapy, because they are too intense and stimulating when used with essential oils. If you are not a massage therapist, you can just work the oils into the skin in a gentle rhythmic motion. The essences can also be used very effectively in reflexology. Different oils can be chosen to correspond with the different areas of the foot.

Madame Maury was mainly responsible for introducing massage as the primary method of working essential oils into the body. She was concerned about their internal use without the supervision of a physician, and set about to find another way. In her book[1] she states:

> If we could make the odoriferous matter penetrate directly through the skin into the extra-cellular spaces and thus into the organic liquids in which the cells bathe; if we could diffuse this fluid matter within a reasonable time and at a reasonable rhythm, it would be possible to establish a new treatment and find a new way.

Never apply pure essential oils to the skin. They must be diluted in a suitable carrier oil. For aromatherapy massage, we usually use a one and a half to three percent dilution of essential oil. Sometimes, as for elderly people, pregnant women, and extremely sensitive people, we use a one half to one percent dilution. Don't be tempted to exceed this; more is not necessarily better. I have found that sometimes the weaker dilutions are even more effective. In general, it is better to start with a weaker mixture and work your way up as you come to know your client and how he or she responds to the oils.

To prepare a percentage dilution, five milliliters (ml) of carrier oil equals 100 drops, so to get an n percent dilution, just add n drops of essential oil to five ml of carrier oil. For example, one drop/five ml will make a one percent dilution, two drops/five ml, two percent, and three drops/five ml, three percent. For those readers more comfortable with ounces, to make a three percent dilution you would add 18 drops of essential oil to one ounce of carrier oil. (One ounce is just over 30 ml.)

Do not use lanolin or mineral carrier oils. Lanolin coats the skin, making it difficult for the essential oils to penetrate, and some people are allergic to it. Mineral oil is a petroleum-based product; it can cause skin dehydration and block the pores.

Always use a vegetable oil, cold-pressed if possible, as a carrier. A good aromatherapy blend should have no other additives. Once blended, your massage oil should have a shelf life of about six months. If you would like it to keep longer, you can add wheatgerm oil, which is an antioxidant.

Here are some suitable carrier oils:

Almond: emollient and nourishing.

Apricot kernel: a good facial oil; absorbs well.

Peach kernel: a good facial oil; absorbs well.

Avocado: nourishing for dry and mature skin; aids penetration.

Jojoba: closest to the skin's natural sebum; fine texture.

Grapeseed: light, fine-textured; excellent all-purpose massage oil.

Wheatgerm: rich in vitamin E; nourishing and scar-reducing.

The following are some massage oil recipes. The amount of essential oil given is per one ounce of carrier oil.

Stimulating
juniper 4 drops
ginger 2 drops
rosemary 8 drops
peppermint 2 drops

Muscular aches and pains
marjoram 6 drops
lavender 6 drops
rosemary 6 drops

Sedative

sandalwood 4 drops
lavender 8 drops
clary sage 6 drops

Ideally, aromatherapy blends should be mixed individually at the time of use. A good therapist will do this, because the client's mood and circumstances vary from day to day. If you make up an ounce at a time, you will have enough to use in the massage, and the remainder can be given to the client for home use.

One benefit of sending clients home with their little bottles with the oils marked on the label is that they continue to use the oils at home and begin to associate particular benefits with particular oils. For example, one of my clients now asks for orange when she feels jaded and needs some joy in her life.

For a healthy person with a relatively toxin-free body, 3 to 6 hours are needed for the oils to fully penetrate into the body. Obese clients, or those with a congested system, may require up to 24 hours for full penetration. If possible, it is better for a client not to bathe for 24 hours after an aromatherapy massage.

Inhalation

Steam inhalation is a good way to treat respiratory and skin problems, and is also useful for altering moods or emotional states. The method consists of adding a few drops of essential oils to a bowl of hot water, then covering the head with a towel and inhaling the aromatic vapors for one to ten minutes. Note that this is not a good method if you have broken capillaries in your face.

For asthmatic people, a better method is to sprinkle a drop of diluted oil on the palm of the hand, rub the hands briskly to create heat, and then cup the hands over the face. This dry method of inhalation is also good for a quick pick-me-up, or if you are someplace where moist inhalation is impossible.

Two or three drops of essential oil are usually enough for an inhalation. Be careful with peppermint, spice, and citrus oils; they are strong and can burn the skin and eyes. One or two drops of these is enough.

Inhalation is a simple and effective way of using essential oils. Madame Maury described inhalation's effect on a girl with a swollen face and congested skin:

> The effect was achieved in a few minutes. The swelling in her face abated before our eyes. It was surprising, one might say spectacular. [2]

The effects of inhalations are swift, but transitory, so it is important to use them regularly, two or three times a day, and back them up with another method such as massage. Inhalations are particularly effective for treating stubborn sinus problems.

Here are some recipes for inhalations:

Headache/migraine
marjoram 1 drop
lavender 1 drop
peppermint 1 drop

Expectorant/lung antiseptic
sandalwood 1 drop
tea-tree 1 drop
benzoin 1 drop

Head colds or blocked sinuses
eucalyptus 1 drop
lavender 1 drop
peppermint 1 drop

Make sure you have plenty of tissues nearby; I've seen these sinus inhalations induce serious drainage problems.

Facial steam
camomile 2 drops
lavender 1 drop

Compresses

Compresses are an old and very good method of applying essential oils to a specific area of the body. They can be hot or cold, depending on the situation. A hot compress should be as hot as bearable, and for a cold compress, put ice cubes in the water. Hot compresses are usually used to reduce muscular and rheumatic pain, to draw out boils and splinters, to relieve menstrual cramps, earache, toothache, etc. Cold compresses are good for sprains, swelling, headache, and to reduce fever. Alternating hot and cold compresses help speed healing in pulled muscles and strained ligaments.

Compresses can also be used to aid the absorption of essential oil applied with massage to the area of the body needing treatment. For example, you could apply an expectorant chest rub, then a compress. Bandaging may be used to hold a compress in place for overnight treatment. This will work because the essences are absorbed into the skin even when the temperature of the compress changes.

To make a compress, add about six drops of essential oil to about a pint of water. Place the material used for the compress into the water, wring it, and apply to the area to be treated. For added effectiveness, an herbal infusion of the same plant can be used instead of water.

Internal Use of Essential Oils

This is an area of much controversy. The French medical service permits the prescription of essences for internal use, much in the same way that a physician in this country would prescribe antibiotics. They are carefully prepared medications, usually in capsule form, and are formulated to be safe for ingestion.

Taking pure oils in tea, water, or honey is **not** a good idea. There is a real possibility of irritating the stomach lining if used incorrectly or in excess. Although many writers suggest this use, the International Federation of Aromatherapists and the International Society of Professional Aromatherapist in England have strongly advised against it unless under the supervision of a medical doctor, as is the practice in France. Cutaneous absorption of the oils is just as effective and much safer.

To quote Madame Maury, herself a biochemist, "…the responsibility for administering them internally could not be carried out except by a competent doctor."[3] Remember that as little as 15 ml of any essential oil taken internally can be fatal, especially wintergreen and pennyroyal. If a person accidentally ingests a quantity of essential oil, he or she should be given plenty of full-fat milk to drink, and immediate medical attention is required.

Burners and Diffusers

Fumigation probably was the first method of utilizing aromatic materials, and it has been used for thousands of years in the religious and cleansing ceremonies of many cultures. As noted in Chapter 1, it was also used to purify the air during the time of the plague.

Vaporizing essence is much cleaner, since there is no smoke. This method can be extremely effective in killing airborne bacteria, as well as in altering mood. Air sprays can be made very simply by adding a few drops of essential oil to some water in a small spray bottle. This is a wonderful nonchemical air freshener; a few sprays can quickly transform the atmosphere in a room.

It is possible to purchase small candle burners, something like the potpourri burners widely available. To use the burner, simply add water to the small bowl at the top and sprinkle about six drops of essential oil into the water. The candle below heats the water and the oil evaporates.

Diffusers are designed to pump minute droplets of essential oil into the air at high pressure. The oil is not heated, air is the propellant, and small quantities of ozone are produced in the process. This also has an invigorating effect.

Here are some aromatic air recipes:

Calming blend
    lavender 4 drops
    petitgrain 2 drops

Antiseptic blend

pine 2 drops
eucalyptus 2 drops
orange 2 drops

Brain-reviving blend

basil 2 drops
rosemary 2 drops
peppermint 2 drops

Respiratory blend

rosemary 2 drops
tea-tree 2 drops
lavender 2 drops

Meditation blend

frankincense 2 drops
sandalwood 2 drops
cedarwood 2 drops

We have seen that there are many ways of using essential oils, and by combining two or more an amazing variety of individual treatments can be created. In fact, it is possible to create a completely aromatic environment both inside and outside the body. It is this versatility of applications that makes aromatherapy a truly exciting therapeutic tool.

Contraindications

Wonderful as they are, essential oils can be harmful. Some are toxic, or skin irritants, and should not be used regularly. Also, the inappropriate use of oils may put some people at risk.

Epilepsy

Sweet fennel, hyssop, sage, and wormwood (wormwood should not be used at all in aromatherapy) are not safe for people with epilepsy, because they could trigger an attack. Be very careful with rosemary; use it, if at all, in very small doses.

Pregnancy

Basil, clary sage, hyssop, juniper, marjoram, and sage should not be used in pregnancy. They could induce abortion or harm the fetus. Avoid fennel, peppermint, and rosemary for the first three months of pregnancy, and then use cautiously, one percent dilution in massage and only three drops in a bath. These oils are emmenagogues, and their use could induce early labor. **Pennyroyal is absolutely not to be used!** It is a known abortive and women have died from trying to induce abortions with it.

High blood pressure

Rosemary, sage, and red thyme are hypertensive, and should not be used by people with high blood pressure. I would also be very careful with the highly stimulant spice oils.

Skin irritants

Basil, lemon, lemongrass, lemon verbena, melissa, peppermint, thyme, tea-tree, cinnamon leaf, sweet fennel, fir needle (Siberian), parsley seed, and pimento leaf can irritate the skin. Use only three drops in baths, and do not use on anyone with sensitive skin or a tendency towards allergic reactions. If using in massage, dilute to one or two percent.

Photosensitization

Angelica, bergamot, cumin, lemon, lime, orange, and verbena all increase the skin's sensitivity to ultraviolet light. Therefore, one should avoid applying them to the skin before exposure to sunlight or any other source of ultraviolet. This is especially true in high-altitude areas with bright sunshine. Exposure after applying these oils will produce large red burn marks, which may not appear until two or three days later. If you want to use these oils for their therapeutic effects, apply them only to areas of the body which will not be exposed.

Even in dull sunlight, bergamot can cause burns. I once heard about someone who had a massage with bergamot in England and got pigmentation marks a few days later. This is astonishing, since we all know how reluctant the sun is to show its face in England!

Toxic oils

These are not to be used at all: cinnamon bark, clove, mugwort, oregano, pennyroyal, savory, wormwood, and wintergreen. Sage, aniseed, clove bud oil, and hyssop should not be used unless you are a trained and experienced therapist.

When blending oils for a client, it's a good idea to let the person smell the oils. If he or she doesn't like the aroma, it may not be needed at the time, or an allergic reaction may occur. A few people are very sensitive and cannot tolerate these powerful substances. If there is any indication of this, it is best to avoid their use altogether.

The use of oils on children or frail, elderly adults requires very weak dilutions (a half to one percent). For everyone, keep the oils away from the eyes, since they can burn the cornea. If accidental eye contact occurs, immediately flush the eye with whole (not skim) milk. Water will do no good and may even spread the oil.

Do not use essential oils on cancer patients without medical supervision. In all cases, do not use any oil continuously for more than three weeks. If you are treating something over a long term, you can use the oil for three weeks, take a week off, then resume using it. This will increase the effectiveness of the treatment.

Never make any medical claims for the oils; prescribing is unlawful unless you are a licensed physician. Careful, responsible, sensitive use of these substances is imperative. Always err on the side of caution, and never suggest their internal use. Using good quality oils will avoid some of the side effects such as nausea, skin irritation, and allergic reactions that I have seen with cheap, synthetic products.

Endnotes

1. Maury, M. *Marguerite Maury's Guide to Aromatherapy: The Secret of Life and Youth.* Saffron Walden, England: C. W. Daniel, 1989.

2. Ibid.

3. Ibid.

5

The Forgotten Sense

The word aroma, the first five letters of the word aromatherapy, defines one of the principal features of the essential oils. It is the aromatic nature of these substances, along with the effects they have on our brain through our sense of smell, that makes aromatherapy more than just the application of sweet-smelling oils during massage.

Our sense of smell is one of the most widely misunderstood and neglected functions of the human body. This seems strange, because in early man the sense of smell was essential to survival. Museums the world over have artifacts from ancient civilizations in which the most precious materials were used to hold scented delicacies.

In modern society, we pay no attention to training our sense of smell. Part of our neglect of this sense may be connected with a puritanical approach to our bodies and their natural functions, which often produce aromas, and part of it undoubtedly is because our sense of smell has been dulled by the synthetic aromas that surround us, by air pollution, and by the use of harsh antiseptics and drugs. We even breed flowers for their beauty, rather than their fragrance!

I've had many students tell me that they can't stand the scent of rose; it makes them nauseous and irritates the nose. When they smell the real thing, they don't even recognize it! Its sad that a synthetic scent has almost totally replaced experience of this heavenly flower.

In teaching aromatherapy, I am constantly amazed by how much education the nose needs to develop the ability to distinguish natural oils from synthetics. A surprising number of my students suffer from "anosmia," loss of the ability to smell.

I believe that by neglecting our sense of smell and therefore the beauty of natural aromas, we have lost much of value. Scent can open areas of subconsciousness and superconsciousness where much knowledge and wisdom is stored—wisdom sorely needed in our culture of extreme rationalism. Perfumes have been seen traditionally as a manifestation of the Deity's love for us. In moments of deep prayer, I have personally experienced a heavenly aroma filling the room and a deep sense of divine love filling my heart.

Jean-Jacques Rousseau said that our sense of smell is imagination itself. Madame Maury saw aromatics as unable to liberate the soul, but felt that by lightening and clearing the mind and emotions, they can help to allow the light of the soul to shine through. And, as Monica Junemann[1] has said, no one can deny that beautiful, natural fragrances awaken our desire to envelop ourselves in life and all it has to offer. Perhaps this is the key to the deeply integrated effect of a good aromatherapy treatment, which heals the body with massage and liberates the soul with a carefully chosen blend of aromatic oils.

Olfaction

The study or science of the sense of smell is called "osmology." If we are to understand how essential oils can affect our mind and emotions, we need to understand the physical mechanisms involved.

Morris[2] calls our sense of smell our "chemical sense of touch" and one of the most important features of this faculty is the direct link between our brain and our environment which occurs in the nose. Only three inches separate the olfactory receptor sites and the brain; the nerve fibers of the olfactory system run directly to the limbic area of the brain without passing through the switching station known as the dorsal thalmus. Olfactory messages also do not pass through the spinal cord, as do most of the other nerve messages in the body. In fact, the two olfactory bulbs are small pieces of the brain which peek out into the environment. Dr. George Dodd, of Warwick University in England, calls the olfactory cells of the nose "brain cells outside the brain." These cells are also the only nerve cells that regenerate, which indicates their importance.

Robert Tisserand has pointed out that the olfactory system is one of the paths we can use to bypass the blood-brain barrier. This is extremely important therapeutically, and shows why we can influence the moods and emotions so quickly and effectively through inhalation of essential oils. Most allopathic drugs (excluding some tranquilizers) have very large molecules and cannot pass through the small capillaries into the brain, which makes the treatment of brain disorders difficult. The direct access offered by olfaction can be a

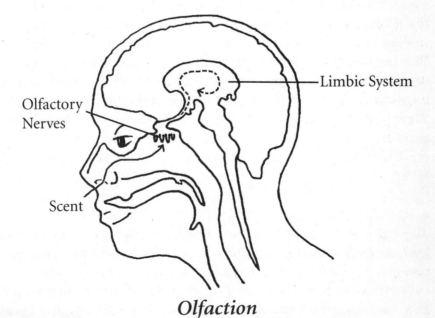

Olfaction

quick and convenient way around this barrier. Cyanide kills in two to three minutes when ingested, in only ten seconds if inhaled.

Let's say that we've opened a bottle of essential oil and held it to our nose for a few minutes, inhaling its exquisite bouquet. Just how is its vapor registered by our brain, and how can this invisible cloud of aroma affect our emotions and hormonal balance so profoundly?

First, the essential oil evaporates and the gaseous substance containing the odoriferous particles enters the nose with the air we breathe. The nose warms the air and the odoriferous particles dissolve in the mucous which covers the olfactory epithelium at the top of the inner nasal cavity. Under the mucous are millions of cilia, tiny hair-like endings of small olfactory nerves which transmit information to one of the two main olfactory nerves.

It is important to remember that the aromatic molecules travel no further than the nose. They trigger a nerve message, and are exhaled. When the cilia detect the presence of the odor molecules, a message is sent along the long axon of the olfactory cells, through the bony plate at the top of the nose, and into the olfactory bulbs, which relay information to the limbic area of the brain. This is a complex area, with 34 structures and 53 pathways, containing subareas linked to the perception of odor (the piriform area), the sensations of pleasure and pain, emotions like rage, fear, sorrow, and sexual feelings. The hippocampus and amygdala areas in the limbic system are specifically related to emotion and memory, and this explains how scent can recall memories and emotions of something that happened a long time ago, like the cheap after-shave your first boyfriend used. Scent memory is much longer-term than visual memory.

The limbic area is one of the oldest parts of the brain, and is called the old brain, also the rhinencephalon, or "smell brain." It is thought to have developed more than 70 million years ago, and predates the cortex, or intellectual brain. Thus through scent we have a direct link to our distant past, and I have long felt that there is much knowledge that we might retrieve if we knew how to use scent correctly. It is also a link to our most distant ancestors and our most basic and animalistic desires. This is evident in the role pheromones play in sexual attraction and mating. In Greek, *pherein* means to bear

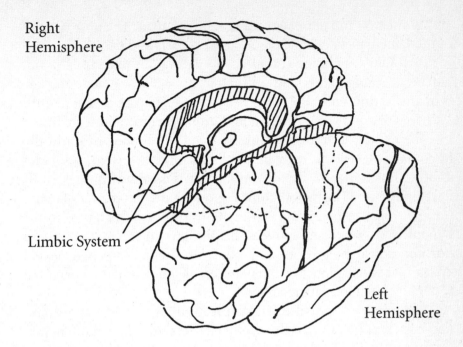

Right
Hemisphere

Limbic System

Left
Hemisphere

Brain Areas

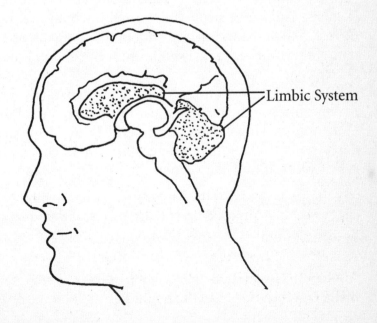

Limbic System

along, or carry, and *hormone* means an excitement. The nose is made of the same type of erectile tissue as the clitoris and penis.

Perfumes containing sexually stimulating oils like sandalwood, patchouli, ylang-ylang, and animal scents act as pheneromes for humans, acting on brain receptors to stimulate the sexual glands. Valerie Worwood[3] has written about aromatherapy and sexuality.

The existence of a close link between the limbic area and the hypothalmus, which regulates the hormonal system, provides another link between sexuality and scent. Tisserand[4] quotes Stoddart as follows: "The hypothalmic region is a major receiver of olfactory neurons, and releases a variety of hormones which pass to the hypophyseal system and induces the pituitary to secrete the suite of hormones which governs and controls the mammalian sexual cycles." We will explore the link between olfaction and the hormonal system in detail in a later chapter.

The limbic system also has connections with the thalmus and neo-cortex, giving aromas the ability to affect conscious thought and reactions. We also know that the essential oils affect the sympathetic and parasympathetic nervous systems.

According to Tisserand,[5] Japanese researcher Torii found that jasmine, ylang-ylang, peppermint, rose, patchouli, neroli, clove, bois de rose, and basil increased activity in the sympathetic nervous system, and marjoram, sandalwood, lemon, chamomile, and bergamot decreased it.

Valnet[6] describes Rovesti's research with patients suffering from nervous diseases, hysteria, and depression. He found that jasmine, sandalwood, orange, ylang-ylang, verbena, and lemon are good for depression, and bergamot, orange blossom, lavender, cypress, lime, rose, violet leaf, and marjoram soothe anxiety. He concluded:

> It may be said that the patients feel as if transported by the essential oil into a different, more agreeable and acceptable world, so that many of their reactive instincts are curbed, and they gradually return towards normality.

Robert Tisserand discusses much of the current research in aromatherapy, behavior, and the brain. Research on the olfactory functions is being done at the Monell Chemical Senses Research Center in Philadelphia, Duke University, the University of Warwick in England, and several Japanese universities.

Implications for Aromatherapy Practice

The implications of the previous paragraphs for holistic aromatherapy are fascinating. The link between scent and psychological/emotional states means that we have a very powerful tool for uniting mind, body, and spirit, and surely this is the basis for true healing.

One of the most obvious implications is that in choosing our blend of oils we must take account of the mental and emotional states of the person with whom we are working. We know that the oils will evaporate during our treatment, even if we do not use an inhalator or diffuser, and they will have non-physical effects. So we can choose oils that are stimulating or calming, oils that promote clear thinking or depress thinking, oils that arouse sexuality or suppress it, oils that are spiritually uplifting, or oils that are grounding.

We can also use oils to stimulate memory, or to help someone recall something that is impeding their personal development. We can help a person to relive a particularly wonderful time of their life, or to reprogram painful associations. For example, we can meditate on a pleasant memory or sensation while inhaling a scent that we associate with a painful area of our past or present. Depression can be lifted with oils we know to have an uplifting effect, and painful emotional situations can be soothed with oils that promote emotional balance. Addictions, frustration, stress, and anger all can be helped.

I know of one aromatherapist who advises his obese clients who are overeating because of depression or loneliness, to inhale an aroma they find particularly pleasing whenever they feel like eating. He finds this "replacement" therapy to be very successful.

Oils can be used in our self-development. We know that aromatic incense and particular scents have been used for spiritual advancement and meditation for thousands of years, in many cultures. Scott Cunningham[7] describes a system of aromatherapy that combines smell and visualization as an agency for growth, change, and self-awareness. He emphasizes inhalation, from diffusers, saturated cotton balls, a bowl of hot water, or in the bath, so massage is not necessary or even desirable when working at this level.

Breathing practices and the development of consciousness have been linked in many systems; it is through our nose that we absorb prana, and our nose is the olfactory gateway to the brain. Certain aromas are known to open pathways to higher consciousness, and since we know that the olfactory sense bypasses the conscious mind, we have much to work with. Advanced spiritual masters are said to sense certain aromas at certain stages of spiritual development. Many healers link physical sickness with soul sickness, so this is another area we need to consider in our work as aromatherapists. This is why it is important to consider the whole person in our consultations and in preparing our blends, because these substances influence us on so many and such subtle levels.

Endnotes

1. Juneman, M. *Enchanting Scents.* Wilmot, Wisconsin: Lotus Press, 1988.

2. Morris, E. *Fragrance.* Greenwich, Connecticut: E. T. Morris & Co., 1984.

3. Worwood, V. *Aromantics.* London: Pan Books, 1987.

4. Tisserand, R. *To Heal and Tend the Body.* Wilmot, Wisconsin: Lotus Press, 1988.

5. Ibid.

6. Valnet, J. *The Practice of Aromatherapy.* Saffron Walden, England: C. W. Daniel, 1980.

7. Cunningham, S. *Magical Aromatherapy.* St. Paul: Llewellyn Publications, 1989.

6

The Breath
of Life

We have already looked at two important ways that the essential oils get into the body: through cutaneous absorption, and through the olfactory system. In discussing the olfactory system, we observed the way the sense of smell operates to influence our psychological and emotional processes. Once we have inhaled the air containing the molecules of essential oil and our olfactory system has perceived the aroma, the air and essential oil molecules continue on through the respiratory system and from there into the circulatory system, and to the particular part of the body where they are needed.

The Process of Respiration

One of the most basic functions of our body is respiration. We inhale and exhale 10-15 times each minute, and although we can live for quite a time without food, we cannot live for more than a few minutes without a continuous supply of fresh air.

All living things breathe the same air, and this unites us in a profound way. The plants we are using in aromatherapy and in phytotherapy also form part of the "lungs" of the planet. In polluting the air and destroying large areas of foliage such as the rain forest, we are in fact jeopardizing the life energy of the earth.

Rowett[1] has defined respiration as "the process whereby oxygen is obtained and used for the oxidation of food materials to liberate energy and produce carbon dioxide and water as waste materials." There is an internal respiration which takes place in each cell to free energy for its growth and various functions. External respiration, with which we are concerned here, is the process whereby oxygen is obtained and carbon dioxide is ejected. The site for this exchange of gases is the lungs. Breathing brings in fresh air, and where essential oils are in use, molecules of essential oils; this air is brought into the lungs, and from the lungs, certain molecules pass into the blood stream and general circulation. In the case of essential oils, this means that through the breath they can reach their various target organs or body system.

Let us imagine we are receiving an aromatherapy massage. Our therapist will apply the oil to our body, and the essential oils will penetrate through our skin and enter the blood stream via the capillaries and intercellular fluid. While we are lying on the table, our therapist will ask us to be conscious of our breathing, and to breathe fully and deeply into relaxation.

In my work as a massage therapist, I have regularly found that the deep breathing and relaxation, along with the essential oils, transports my clients into altered states of consciousness, and about 85 percent fall asleep during the massage. I haven't noticed such total relaxation when essential oils were not used.

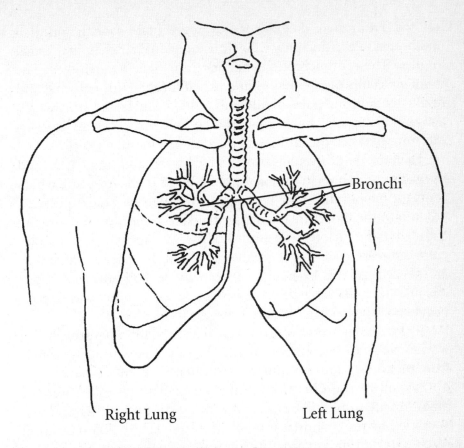

Bronchi

Right Lung　　　Left Lung

Basic Lung Structure

One of our first responses will be to the aroma, and we will begin to feel ourselves relaxing, becoming more alert, etc., depending on the oils chosen by our therapist. Next we will feel the molecules of oil carried up into our nose, where the air will be filtered and warmed by the cilia and mucous membranes lining the nasal passages, and then feel it passing down through our pharynx, larynx, trachea, and into the bronchi of our lungs. We are assuming the use of high quality essential oil, not the synthetic type which stops somewhere in the sinuses and proceeds to give us a headache!

The two main bronchi (one for each lung) divide into finer and finer lobar bronchi. The right lung has three lobes and the left lung has two. From there they divide into segmental bronchi, and then into bronchioles, which serve the little individual air chambers called lobules. These bronchioles subdivide into finer bronchioles. The small molecules of essential oil are carried through this network, and finally these bronchioles divide into alveolar ducts and sacs, which end up in alveoli, small cavities one cell thick, where gaseous exchange between the air in the lungs and the blood takes place.

Each cluster of alveoli is surrounded by very thin capillaries, and the gases and vapors in the air, once dissolved in the moisture which coats the membrane of the alveoli, pass through into the capillaries, go on into the bloodstream, are returned to the heart, and are distributed to the various cells of the body. Thus the essential oil molecules can reach their target organs and the body systems where they are needed. At this exchange between the alveoli and the bloodstream, the capillaries give up carbon dioxide and other waste products to be expelled from the lungs in exhalation.

If the fact that essential oils can reach the bloodstream in this way seems strange, consider anesthesia, or the chemicals we inhale from tobacco, or lead poisoning in children from auto exhaust.

Not all of the essential oil inhaled will necessarily enter the bloodstream; some will be exhaled with the next breath. The oil that is carried by the bloodstream will circulate with the blood until it reaches its destination, does its job, and is finally excreted as waste through the urine, the feces, the lungs, or perspiration.

As an exercise, inhale some essential oil consciously and deeply, and see if you can feel the oil entering your lungs and diffusing through your body. Be aware of any particular area that attracts the oil. Do this with each oil you meet, and record your results.

Essential Oils and
the Respiratory System

We know that there is a group of oils which have a particular affinity for the respiratory system. In this section we will discuss the particular therapeutic properties appropriate to this body system, and look at the oils which are indicated in each case. The main therapeutic properties we are looking for are:

Antiseptics

Valnet[2] describes the incredible antiseptic effect of vaporized essential oils in killing airborne bacteria and organisms; thus we can use essential oils to purify the air before taking it into our lungs.

All essential oils are antiseptic to some extent, but Valnet mentions the following as of particular value when used in a vaporized state: lemon, thyme, orange, bergamot, juniper, clove, citronella, lavender, niaouli, peppermint, rosemary, sandalwood, and eucalyptus. For those of you interested in chemical constituents, these essences appear to have a high content of terpenes. Thus, we can use burners and diffusers to prevent respiratory and other problems before they strike. I know of a day-care center which diffuses oils, and they find that the children have far fewer colds and flu during the winter months.

As far as specific pulmonary antiseptics are concerned, clove is specific to the tuberculosis bacillus, thyme kills the streptococcus and tuberculosis bacilli, garlic is a modifier of bronchial secretions. A blend of pine, thyme, peppermint, lavender, rosemary, cloves, and cinnamon makes a good blend for purification of the air.

Essential oils which are good pulmonary antiseptics are: clove, hyssop, juniper, lavender, lemon, peppermint, pine, rosemary, sandalwood, bergamot, cinnamon, and eucalyptus. Garlic oil is also very good, but most people prefer to take this in capsule form, rather than rub it into their skin. Of course, eating plenty of raw garlic is a good preventative measure during the winter. The lungs are the main site of excretion for garlic oil, so it can work directly on any bacteria there.

Antiviral

Some lung infections are the result of viral infections, and oils such as tea-tree and eucalyptus can be of help here.

Antispasmodic

These oils have the effect of calming spasms in smooth muscle tissue. Good pulmonary antispasmodics are: clary sage, peppermint, thyme, eucalyptus, lavender, and sandalwood.

Antitussive

These oils help soothe coughing. Examples are: hyssop, lavender, eucalyptus, pine, rosemary, and sandalwood. Sandalwood has been repeatedly praised by my clients as a wonderful cough suppressant, allowing many who might cough all night to get a good night's sleep.

Balsamic

Oils such as eucalyptus, pine, and thyme help to soften phlegm so it can be expelled.

Expectorants

Oils which help in the removal of excess phlegm are: benzoin, cedarwood, eucalyptus, hyssop, lemon, myrrh, peppermint, pine, and sandalwood. In England, where many of my clients seemed to have chronic catarrh, I gave them expectorants such as eucalyptus, pine, and sandalwood, and found that this almost invariably helped clear up persistent problems of this kind.

Oils for Specific Respiratory Ailments

Asthma: lavender, marjoram, benzoin, cypress, eucalyptus, pine.

Bronchitis: benzoin, cedarwood, eucalyptus, hyssop, peppermint, rosemary, sandalwood, frankincense, pine, clove.

Emphysema: basil, eucalyptus, thyme, hyssop, garlic.

Hay fever: lavender, camomile, eucalyptus.

Influenza (bronchitic): cinnamon, clove, eucalyptus, lemon, thyme.

Intercostal neuralgia: peppermint.

Laryngitis: benzoin, sandalwood, lavender, sage.

Nosebleeds: lemon.

Pneumonia: eucalyptus, lavender, lemon, pine.

Respiratory stimulant: cinnamon, camphor.

Sinusitis: eucalyptus, lavender, peppermint, lemon, pine, thyme.

Sore throat (also tonsillitis): geranium, lemon, sage, thyme, ginger.

Tuberculosis: eucalyptus, garlic, lemon, pine.

Whooping cough: clary, basil, cypress, hyssop, lavender, rosemary, garlic.

The best methods of application for oils in treating respiratory problems, or in working on getting oils into the body via the respiratory system are: inhalations, chest and spinal massage, compresses, and diffusers and burners. Baths create a lot of vaporized essences, and, as mentioned earlier, all exposure to essential oils results in some inhalation of the vapors.

If you study the list of essential oils used to treat respiratory problems, you will find that they come from a fairly small range of plants. Many of them are trees: leaves, resins, and woods, and of course, the all-time favorite is eucalyptus. One school of thought suggests using the leaf oils for acute and short-term imbalances of the respiratory system, and the woods and resins for more chronic conditions. Generally, the woods and resins tend to be more drying and soothing, while the leaves are more stimulant and active in fighting pulmonary bacteria.

Another view of the essential oils which can benefit the respiratory system is put forward by Dietrich Gumbel.[3] He believes that the oils from the leaves of the plant have a direct relationship to the function of the lungs, since they are the respiratory organs for the plants, and indirectly for the earth itself. During the day they absorb carbon dioxide from the air and give off oxygen and water, which we need to take into our lungs in respiration.

The Emotional Basis of
Respiratory Disorders

Some breathing and respiratory problems such as hyperventilation, shortness of breath, and rapid breathing are caused by underlying nervous and emotional problems, so you will need to look deeper to determine the cause of the disorder. Asthma is another condition which has been linked to emotional factors as well as heredity.

When you are working with someone it is always a good idea to observe their breathing patterns. This can tell you much about their inner state. In many Eastern healing traditions, the breath is of the essence, the source of life-giving *prana,* and many systems of breathing practice have developed in various spiritual disciplines.

Breathing can be used in centering, meditation, visualization, directing energy around the body, relaxation, and so forth, so we can use it consciously in addition to the unconscious breathing we automatically do. Knowledge of the breath can be of immense help in our work as therapists, and it is important to take time to explore this application of our oils.

Before you begin work with anyone, whether it is a consultation, massage, or even giving a talk, it is a good idea to center your attention on your breathing. Taking several long, deep breaths will calm your mind, energize your physical and subtle bodies, and allow you to become more aware of the energies within and around you.

You may wish to combine this conscious breathing with some imagery, such as imagining you are breathing in a healing color, with a particular oil that you find appropriate to the work at hand, an affirmation or prayer, or an imagery you particularly like, such as surrounding yourself with a halo of protective light.

When you approach the client or friend you are going to massage and are centered, take a moment to observe his or her breathing patterns. Notice the quality and intensity of the inhalation and exhalation, and whether one element of breathing is dominant. Sudden and forced inhalation can indicate anger, anxiety, or fear; shallow, gentle, and gradual inhalation can denote tiredness, gloom, depression. Sometimes the person may not even seem to be breathing.

As I work on massage clients, I continue to watch the breathing pattern change. When the work has finally released some long-held emotional pattern or physical imbalance, almost always a deepening and opening of the breathing occurs, or a long sigh, as if the client is relieved to finally let go of that particular burden. I like to see this happen, because it makes me feel that we are making progress in our working together.

I often ask a client to join me in some slow, deep breathing before I start a treatment, and request that he or she exhale all tension, fear, and sadness before we start, so that we are ready to accomplish some healing together. I usually wait until our breathing is synchronized, and I feel the emptying taking place, to start treatment. During the treatment, it is also useful to ask the client to direct his or her breath to certain areas of the body at certain times, or to alter his or her breathing as you stretch, or apply pressure to certain points. Different types of breath work have been developed. Because of the nature of the essential oils and how they enter through breathing, this certainly would be something worth exploring.

The yoga science of breathing, *Pranayama,* is solely concerned with the quality of the breath and the pattern of inhalation, exhalation, and suspension, which we can learn to control for specific purposes. We can increase our intake of prana, direct that more efficiently, prepare our consciousness for meditation, relax and control the mind and emotions, and cleanse and stabilize the circulation, lungs, and nervous system.

The use of aromatics also helps us to achieve deeper breathing. When we smell something beautiful we open up to it, want to inhale it deeply, and become aware of our breath. Along with partaking of the healing power of the oil, we take in more oxygen, and more life force from the environment, and this nourishes us on all levels, physically, mentally, emotionally, and spiritually.

Alternatively, when we smell something foul, our instinct is to stop breathing, to refuse to allow this offensive substance to enter our being, and thus we reduce our intake of oxygen and prana. This ultimately leads to inefficient functioning of our body systems, and illness. The effects of pollution, offensive surroundings, and lack of fresh air thus affect our health in many subtle ways. We literally close off to life, and this closure starts with the fact that we allow our environment to become so polluted in the first place. The breath is food to the spirit in more ways than one.

Endnotes

1. Rowett, H. *Basic Anatomy and Physiology.* London: John Murray, 1959.

2. Valnet, J. *The Practice of Aromatherapy.* Saffron Walden, England: C. W. Daniel, 1980.

3. Gumbel, G. *Principles of Holistic Skin Therapy with Herbal Essences.* Heidelberg: Haug, 1986.

7

The Body's Envelope

Aromatherapy skin care is one of the most interesting uses of essential oils. It is, of course, an entire specialty of its own, but in this chapter we will discuss the structure and functions of the skin, skin types, skin problems, the ways in which the essential oils affect the skin, and some simple recipes for making your own aromatherapy skin care products.

The Structure and Function of the Skin

The skin consists of three main layers: the epidermis, the dermis, and the superficial fascia, or subcutaneous layer. It is the largest organ of the body, weighs about four kilograms, and is thinnest on the face, eyelids, and lips, thickest on the palms and soles. The skin is composed of compound epithelial tissue, laid on a foundation of fibrous connective tissue, into which it interlocks by a series of finger-like projections called papillae.

The Epidermis

This is the outer layer of the skin, and is made up of five sublayers, in which the transformation from basal cells with well-defined nuclei to dead cells with no nuclei takes place. The five sublayers are:

The stratum corneum or horny layer

This consists of dead, flattened cells in which the cytoplasm and nucleus have been replaced by the protein keratin. These cells are constantly shed and replaced by new cells from the basal layer beneath. They contain a fatty material which keeps the skin watertight and helps to protect the skin from bacterial invasion. This is the surface of the skin that we see. Skin brushing and using a loofah help to remove the dead cells that are ready to be shed, and stimulate the circulation needed to nourish new cell growth.

I have observed that a 15–20 minute soak in a bath with essential oils added seems to lift the dead skin cells from the surface. Exfoliants used in skin therapy are aimed at removing dead cells which are ready to be shed; these can harbor oil and bacteria if allowed to build up on the skin.

Stratum lucidum or transparent layer

This sublayer is only a few cells thick and is thought to be a barrier zone which controls the transmission of water through the skin. At this level, the cells have lost their clear boundaries and the nuclei are becoming indistinct.

Stratum granulosum or granular layer

This sublayer consists of several layers of flattened spindle-shaped cells which have lost their nuclei and contain a number of granules which contain a substance called keratohyaline. It is in this sublayer

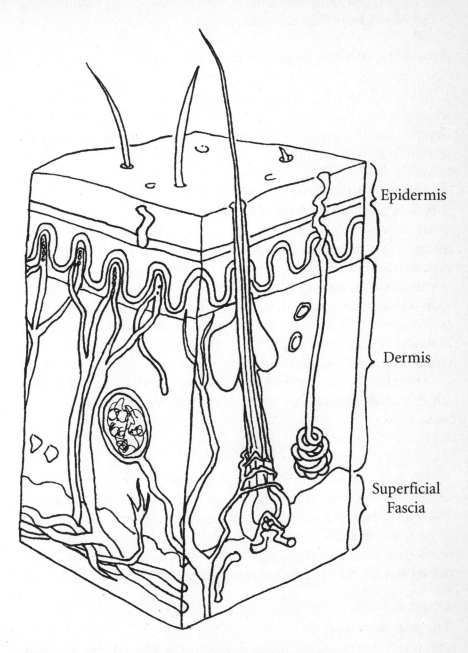

Epidermis

Dermis

Superficial
Fascia

The Layers of the Skin

that the process of keratinization, which is the change from living cells to dead, horny flat cells takes place.

Stratum spinosum, prickle layer, or mucosum

These are the cells which lie above the basal or germinative level. Because they are relatively young, they have not yet lost their nuclei. The cells are still well-defined, polygonal, and connected to each other by fine threads filled with tissue fluid, forming interlinked projections with a spiky appearance.

Stratum germinativum or basal layer

This is the deepest sublayer of the epidermis, and it is here that the birth of new cells takes place. The new cells push the old cells towards the surface, and the nourishment needed for the constant reproduction of cells comes from the capillary blood vessels in the dermis. Skin rejuvenation takes place at this level, and many things such as age, diet, circulation, exposure to heat, cold, light, drugs, smoking, etc. will influence the rate of cell regeneration. The average life cycle of each new cell is about six weeks. Therefore, any skin treatment aimed at improving the skin will need at least six weeks to two months before any real improvement can be expected. Oils which are cytophilactic are said to stimulate new cell growth.

The Dermis

This is the major layer which lies beneath the epidermis, and here are found the collagen and elastin fibers which give the skin tensile strength and elasticity, the sweat and sebaceous glands, hair follicles, arrector pili muscles, lymphatic vessels, nerve endings, arteries, and veins. This layer contains a high water content, and dehydration at this level may cause premature aging effects on the skin. The dermis has two sublayers:

The papillary layer

This is the interface with the epidermis, where all of the protrusions and irregularities called papillae are found. Many nerve endings of touch are found in this layer, as are the fine capillaries and veins which bring nourishment and oxygen to the skin, carry away waste products, and provide blood to the epidermis.

The reticular layer

Many sweat and sebaceous glands are found here, along with the collagen and elastic fibers which give the skin its elasticity. These elastic qualities diminish with age, as can be seen in the lack of firm skin tone in the elderly. Nerves concerned with the sensations of touch, deep pressure, pain, heat, and cold are found in this layer, as are the arrector pili muscles.

The Superficial Fascia

This is the bottom skin layer, which separates the dermis from the muscles, allowing the skin to move freely over the underlying structures. It is composed of elastic fibers, fibrous tissue, and fatty tissue. The fat tissue is a cushion for the nerve endings and blood vessels in the dermis and provides protection against the loss of body heat.

Skin Functions

Now that we have some idea of the structure of the skin, we need to understand its five principal functions:

Temperature control

Much of the body's heat is distributed around the body by the circulatory system. The control of temperature can occur through the expansion and contraction of the superficial capillaries. It is also affected by the evaporation of perspiration from the surface of the skin. Increased production of sweat reduces body temperature and decreased production increases it. Stimulant oils can be used to increase the body heat through stimulation of the circulation, there are also oils which help with dilation and constriction of the blood vessels.

We all know the warming effect of a hot bath on a cold winter's night. Adding "warming" oils such as cinnamon, marjoram, ginger, or rosemary can substantially increase the effect by stimulating blood circulation. The husband of one of my English students was a "busker" on the streets of London. Before he set out for a day's work in the damp English weather, he would have a rubdown with black pepper oil. He said this changed his life, since the hot massage seemed to keep him warm all day, and he played his fiddle with a new exuberance.

Protection

The skin is protected from bacterial invasion and absorption of water by the horny layer. The fat layer also protects against water and loss of body fluids. The melanin content of the epidermis protects the body from absorption of ultraviolet and infrared rays. Vitamin D is formed by exposure to sunlight, and this nourishes the bones. The skin is continually exposed to bacteria, and a number of means of dealing with them exist. If the skin's natural defenses fail, infections, boils, or other skin disorders can result. One of the ways the skin protects itself is its acid mantle. The acidic nature of the fluid on the outer surface of the skin helps to neutralize bacteria. Sebum is bacteriostatic, bactericidal, and fungicidal. It also lubricates the skin and helps to maintain an intact skin surface. Sweat is also bactericidal when not present in excessive amounts. Essential oils can help the protective function by virtue of their antiseptic, bactericidal, antifungal, and anti-inflammatory properties.

Absorption

Because the skin is designed to prevent the absorption of harmful substances into the body, only certain substances can pass through it. The determining factor is molecular size. It is thought that the primary routes for substances to enter are through the sebaceous gland openings, hair follicles and the skin itself (to a limited extent). One of the main reasons that essential oils can penetrate the skin is their small molecular size. Substances such as lanolin and mineral oil, often found in so-called aromatherapy products, have a large molecular size and so will not be absorbed. Massage can aid absorption of the essential oils. It is useful to remember that the skin cannot absorb while it is excreting. Infrared heat can be used before application of the oils, to help open the pores and aid absorption, as can hot towels and massage in a facial. Hot steam, which increases the perspiration of the skin, should be avoided if essential oils are to be applied directly afterwards. I've often noted that the application of a fair amount of essential oils, as in massage, results in a faint scent of the oil in sweat or urine excreted a few hours after the massage.

Excretion and secretion

Excretion is the elimination of waste products through the skin, and normally one quarter of the body's waste products and some excess water are disposed of in this way. Inefficiency in this function puts a burden on the other three organs of elimination: the kidneys, lungs, and bowels. Alternatively, if these organs are not functioning efficiently, the skin takes over some of their work, and this can give rise to congested or edematous skin, boils, rashes, and other skin problems. A clear skin will reflect relatively clean body systems, and any skin treatment should approach skin imbalances in an holistic way, looking at the body and its functions as a whole.

Secretion refers to the production of substances by the cells and glands of the skin. A good example is sebum, which is produced by the oil glands to keep the skin supple. Essential oils can be used to help balance the secretion of the glands; for example, dry skin produces too little sebum, while oily skin produces too much. We also know that essential oils can be helpful as hormonal balancers, and this will have an effect on the skin. My experience in skin care has shown that the regular application of essential oils will definitely rebalance the skin over a period of time, so that many clients have a marked change in skin type. In fact, some even achieve the "normal" skin condition, which usually is rarely found in adults.

Sensation

The skin provides the barrier between the outer and the inner, the world and ourselves. The sensory nerves in the skin allow us to experience and respond to our environment. Skin is the organ of touch, which is one of the most powerful and important of our senses, emotionally, psychologically, and physically. Touch is very important to us as aromatherapists, and it is through skin contact that we can understand much about our clients' state of balance or imbalance, their temperature, the state of their nervous system, tissues, muscles, and so forth.

Our emotional state is reflected in our skin. Poor skin may not necessarily represent poor living habits, but may be telling a story of stress, anxiety, lost love, spiritual crisis, or any other problem. In such cases, the oils could be used to help soothe the underlying disease on the emotional, psychological, or spiritual level. For example, rose would be useful for a woman who had just lost her husband. Her skin may need this oil, but it may not, in which case you could give her massages with rose, and make another facial oil for her to use at home. You could also add rose to the facial oil, or use it in a facial massage if it were not contra indicated by her facial condition.

The sensory receptors of the skin respond to pain, touch, pressure, and temperature. Note which are located in the epidermis and which are found deeper in the dermis. These receptors play a vital role in connecting us with our environment, enabling us to respond to it. Think about how massage could trigger these receptors.

A good example is a client who came to me about six weeks before her wedding. She normally had beautiful skin, but during the past few weeks her skin had become very sensitive, blotchy, and blemished. She had a good diet and skin-care routine, so I suspected that stress was a significant factor. I chose oils to relieve the stress, such as calming lavender, rose for the emotional upheaval, and neroli for the anxiety. These oils were also appropriate for her delicate English skin. She had weekly facials and by the time her wedding date arrived, she had beautiful skin and was calm and radiant.

The Classification of Skin Types

There is a generally accepted method of skin classification according to the balance of water and sebum in the tissues. Each category actually represents a state of imbalance; the perfect or normal skin is hard to find. Essential oils can be used to help correct the particular imbalances represented by the skin types.

Normal Skin

Few adults have normal skin, which is evenly balanced in oil and moisture content. This is the skin of prepubescence or childhood, and is smooth, free of blemishes, firm, finely textured, with no enlarged pores, unwrinkled, soft, and velvety. The other skin types can be seen as deviations from this ideal, and all methods of skin rejuvenation are attempts to return the skin to this state.

Dry Skin

This skin type is characterized by a fine texture, with no apparent pores, and often has superficial wrinkles or lines. If extremely dry, it may become flaky, can be sensitive, itchy, and feel tight and stretched after washing. This type of skin is often the first to age, and it needs a constant replenishment of moisture and oil. Its main cause is inadequate production of sebum and the resulting inability to trap surface moisture. The output of sebum also decreases with age, so skin generally gets drier with time. Other factors leading to this condition are hormonal imbalance, inadequate intake of vitamin C and oil in the diet, harsh treatment with soap, astringents, too much sun, central heating, and dry climactic conditions.

Aromatherapy skin care is really very simple, and is based on the age-old routine of cleanse, tone, and moisturize. For cleaning, use a bland, non-scented lotion with no lanolin or mineral oil, and as few emulsifiers and preservatives as possible. Almond or jojoba oil makes a good cleanser. For toning, use simple floral waters or infusions, and then the facial oil appropriate to your skin type. Once or twice a week use an exfoliant and a mask.

Essential oils

The balancers, lavender and geranium, can also be used for oily skin, as they are thought to help balance sebum and general hormonal production. Camomile, rose, neroli, and jasmine are good for the sensitivity, irritation, and flakiness that often accompanies dry skin. Camomile and rose also are useful for thread veins. Benzoin and calendula are good for cracked skin, skin exposed to the wind, chapped skin, psoriasis, eczema, and dermatitis. Sandalwood and patchouli help with fluid and sebum levels.

Carrier oils

Avocado, almond, wheatgerm, jojoba, or apricot kernel are good carrier oils for dry skin treatment. Please note that like the essential oils, carrier oils have different properties, and using the correct carrier oils makes a big difference in your facial blends.

Facial tonics

Rose water or camomile infusion.

Masks

Avocado pulp or egg yolk.

Dry skin treat

Gently massage chosen facial oil blend, apply hot towels and let oils soak in under the towels for 20 minutes. Generally, make your facial oils with one to three percent essential oil. For people with sensitive skin, start with a low percentage and work your way up. This is particularly true of some of the stronger oils like rosemary.

Oily Skin

This type of skin generally is shiny, has open pores, may have a sallow or dingy color, has a tendency to blackheads, and is generally seen in younger persons. It's greasy as a result of over-production of sebum; there is an unevenness of texture, and often excessive skin acidity. Other contributing factors are bad diet, metabolic disorders, hormonal imbalances, insufficient skin hygiene, or using harsh preparations which strip the oil from the skin, causing it to go into over-production.

The essential oils can help balance sebaceous production and also act as antiseptics and natural astringents. The proper carrier oil can be used on oily skin, although it may seem strange. Remember, the essential oils penetrate the surface and balance the skin from the inside out. In this way, they are different from preparations which strip the oil from the surface or are simply harsh antiseptics.

A good example of this was John, in his late twenties with a history of acne all of his teenage years. His skin care had comprised all of the usual harsh alcohol-based, strongly antiseptic products marketed to teenagers. He had also tried antibiotics.

I spent an afternoon giving him a facial using a mild natural cleansing lotion, steam with essential oils, a facial massage using ylang-ylang, lemon, and peppermint, and a simple mud mask. I instructed him to do the full routine once a week, and gave him a toner and a facial lotion using the same oils to apply after cleansing his face twice a day with the mild cleanser—not soap. Within six weeks his skin was clear, and the only trace of his acne was the scarring left by his years of suffering from ineffective treatment.

It is important with this skin type to keep the body systems as clean as possible, so lots of water, fresh fruits and vegetables are important, with less emphasis on red meat, fatty food, refined sugar, coffee, tea, and alcohol.

Essential oils

Lavender, geranium and ylang-ylang are sebum balancers. Bergamot, lemon, juniper, are antiseptics. Cypress and juniper are astringents and help with fluid levels. Rosemary is a circulatory stimulant and detoxifier. Lemongrass helps with dilated pores and poor skin tone.

Many oils can be used, but remember that for facial application, they must be pleasant-smelling and not too strong or irritating. With some of the stronger oils, such as cypress and juniper, I would begin with a one percent dilution and work upwards.

Carrier oils

Jojoba, grapeseed, wheatgerm, hazelnut oil, soya oil, and carrot oil.

Toners

Orange flower water, witch hazel, peppermint, lavender, or thyme infusion.

Masks

Deep cleansing two or three times a week is especially important for this skin type. Use an exfoliant regularly to stimulate circulation and remove toxins and use a face mask regularly. The mask also helps to stimulate circulation and deep cleanse the skin. Clays such as kaolin and fuller's earth make a good base for this mask. You can mix with yogurt, cucumber pulp, and a drop of essential oil.

Combination Skin

This type of skin is a mixture of dry skin with oily patches on the T-zones, where the sebaceous glands are most prevalent, the forehead, nose, and chin. Generally, it is best to treat each area separately, using the appropriate oils and masks.

Essential oils

Geranium and lavender can be used on both areas, and can help balance this type of skin.

Normal, dry, oily, and combination are the four main skin classifications, but the following are additional skin types which you will encounter:

Sensitive Skin

More and more people seem to have skin sensitivities and allergies, particularly to the chemicals and perfumes in many skin care products. Most of these people can use essential oils with no problems, but please do a patch test before using them on a large area, and stick to low dilutions. This type of skin is usually very fine, and reacts quickly to the touch, with redness or rashes. It is often prone to eczema and dermatitis. People with this skin type are often very sensitive and finely tuned physically and emotionally.

Essential oils

Camomile is anti-inflammatory, soothing, good for rashes, redness, and eczema. Rose is very gentle and tonic. Benzoin heals irritated skin and is good for dermatitis. Avoid soap and lanolin on this skin type, because they can often trigger a reaction. Also stay away from any oils which could be too stimulating, like ginger and citrus oils. This is true for the skin all over the body, not just on the face. Start with one essential oil at a time and test the skin's reaction before making a blend. Oils other than the three noted above can be used on this skin type when they have been tested individually.

Carrier oils

Jojoba, apricot kernel, almond, aloe vera gel.

Toners

Rose water, Evian water, camomile infusion.

Masks

Pulverized oatmeal mixed with a little rose water.

Edematous Skin

This skin type is characterized by an excess of fluid. This can be due to an hormonal imbalance, metabolic disturbances, poor circulation, or poor lymphatic drainage. Edematous skin often feels cold to the touch, and there is puffiness, particularly around the eyes. It also chaps easily, and is prone to chilblains.

Essential oils

Geranium and lavender for hormonal balance. Juniper, geranium, cypress, and fennel for diuretic qualities. Rosemary increases circulation and reduces toxins.

Carrier oils
Jojoba, grapeseed, almond.

Toners
Infusion of fennel or rosemary, Evian water, rose water.

Masks
Pulped tomato or strawberries.

Facial massage should be done in the direction of the lymph nodes to help drain the excess fluid. Lymphatic massage can also be done, as can whole body massage on a regular basis.

Dehydrated Skin

This type of skin may have enough oil, but lacks moisture. The texture of this skin may be like very fine orange peel, with itchiness and flaking. Lack of water in the tissues can be caused by insufficient fluid intake, poor lymphatic functioning, dieting, climactic conditions, central heating, or lack of sebum. Drinking lots of water is important with this type of skin.

Essential oils
Camomile for irritation. Neroli is soothing and rejuvenating. Sandalwood, patchouli, geranium, orange, and fennel help regulate the fluid balance in the body. Palmarosa is a hydrating oil.

Carrier oils
Hazelnut, avocado, jojoba, spray of Evian water.

Toners
Orange flower water, apple juice.

Masks
Cucumber pulp, slices of cucumber, or yogurt and honey.

Mature or Aging Skin

This type of skin is extra dry, lacks both oil and moisture, is developing wrinkles and lines, especially around the eyes and mouth, could be aging prematurely due to exposure to sun, wind, and harsh climactic conditions.

This skin is also losing elasticity and firmness, with underlying fat shrinking and skin loosening. This is not seen so much in women who are overweight, because the excess fat helps support the skin. One of the things that has most convinced me of the efficacy of essential oils in rejuvenating the skin is the lovely skin and youthful appearance of the "grand dames" of aromatherapy whom I have met. Every one of them has skin that looks years younger than would be expected. Their skin is clear, with few wrinkles and a beautiful texture. I'm sure that none of them has had a face-lift.

One of my colleagues, a nurse, reports great success in healing radiation burns induced by cancer treatment, using essential oils such as neroli and lavender. This confirms the regenerative qualities of the oils.

Essential oils

Frankincense, neroli, and lavender. These are all known as cytophilactic oils; they stimulate the production of new cells in the basal layer. They are also called rejuvenating oils. Clary sage, cypress, and fennel are plant estrogens which help during menopause. Geranium is a general balancer for all unbalanced skin. Benzoin, jasmine, and myrrh soothe dry, cracked, rough skin. Myrrh is rejuvenating, as well. Lemon is good for wrinkles. Rose is a gentle tonic for firmer skin texture, and, along with camomile, is good for thread veins.

Carrier oils

Avocado, jojoba, wheatgerm, almond, borage, carrot, evening primrose, peach, or almond kernel.

Toners

Rose water, Evian water spray, lavender, or rose infusion.

Masks

Avocado pulp and honey mixed with finely ground almonds. Yogurt for crepey skin and dull, dingy necks.

Acne

This is more complicated than oily skin, and is often seen in young people when the skin imbalance may be caused by hormonal imbalances. I have also seen a lot of acne in women in their thirties, probably because their hormones are starting to change. Some women also have premenstrual acne due to hormonal imbalance.

Acne vulgaris is characterized by greasy skin, caused by increased output of sebum. The skin color is generally sallow, with blackheads, papules, and pustules often present. It may involve the face, chest, back and shoulders, or may be confined to only one of these areas. The color of blackheads results from the blockage of the hair follicle by a plug of keratin, which is darkened by the pigment melanin. Sometimes a secondary staphylococcal infection is present, and pimples and inflammation form around the blackhead.

This infection may involve the sebaceous gland, and a deep-seated condition can become established. Extensive acne can cause deep scarring; early treatment and control of the spread of the pustules is important if this is to be avoided. Acne often clears up with age, but much can be done to minimize its spread.

Essential oils

Lemongrass is an astringent good for open pores. Lemon and bergamot are antiseptics and astringents. Lavender is a sebum balancer, antiseptic, and cytophilactic. Carrot for vitamin A content. Camomile is an anti-inflammatory agent. Cedarwood is antiseptic and slightly astringent. Clary sage and frankincense are cell regenerators. Cypress is an astringent and tonic. Geranium is a tonic, revitalizer, and balancer of sebum. Juniper is a decongestant and detoxifier. Neroli is cytophilactic and soothing. Peppermint is a decongestant. Rosemary is antiseptic and decongestant. Tea-tree helps the immune system.

Oils should be chosen according to what you are trying to accomplish. At first, you might use antiseptic, anti-inflammatory, and astringent oils. When the spots are clearing, you might change to regenerating and balancing oils, and introduce carriers like wheatgerm to help with the scarring and the generation of new cells.

Cleansing is extremely important with acne, and a gentle, natural cleansing lotion is best. Harsh cleansers and soap can make the skin worse by stripping off all of the natural oil and stimulating the skin to make more and more sebum.

Skin should be cleansed two or three times a day. If the spots are not infected, a gentle exfoliant can be used. Massage should be kept to a minimum. Compresses using some of the oils listed above are comforting and useful, depending on what you are trying to do.

Carrier oils
Jojoba, wheatgerm (for vitamin E to help with scarring), almond, evening primrose, borage seed. Oils can be added to a bland, all-vegetable lotion which you might be able to find in a health store.

Toners
Diluted cider vinegar, lavender-bergamot tonic, Evian water spray (the skin still needs moisture), witch hazel.

Masks
Kaolin or fuller's earth mixed with a little herbal infusion (see oily skin), cabbage water, or pulverized grapes. You can also add a drop of essential oil of your choice.

Diet is especially important, and vitamins A and E can help. Full body massage with detoxifying oils such as fennel, rosemary, or juniper can help, as can lots of fresh air, exercise, and sun in moderation. The emotional anguish this condition causes should also be addressed, and relaxing oils such as lavender can help with this. These oils can also be used in the bath.

Eczema

This is one of the most distressing conditions, and while I am sure that my own long-standing eczema was cured by essential oils, it is difficult to treat, because there are so many individual factors to consider. Eczema is characterized by an itching red area with pin-sized vesicles, which progresses to scaly, dry patches, sometimes with "weeping." It involves the epidermis and upper layers of the dermis, and can be caused by contact with an external allergen, or internal stimulus via the bloodstream. Allergies, hay fever, and asthma seem linked to it; this combination of conditions seems to run in families. It is usually connected with sensitive skin, and is often stress-related.

I suffered with eczema for about 25 years, and tried cortisone, diet, vitamins, and anything else that was thought to help. Sometimes my legs would get so bad that I'd have to bandage them. The outbreaks were usually related to stressful, particularly emotional periods in my life, and I despaired of ever getting rid of the affliction.

After using essential oils regularly for a long time, I finally licked it, and have been completely free of eczema for at least five years. I believe the oils worked on many levels. Merely applying the oils locally helped. They also seem to have helped me deal with stress, physically and emotionally; I don't have the mood swings that I used to have.

I was recently the subject of a feature story in a local newspaper, which mentioned my success with eczema. This produced a flood of letters from people who suffer from this miserable condition. One particular case stood out.

This man had suffered for 50 years, had tried everything, had participated in university studies, traveled all over to find help, and still had it! He had a job where he dealt with the public, and was very conscious of his skin, which created additional stress. He also suffered from many allergies. He started using various essential oils in a bland, vegetable-based, unscented lotion, and for the first time his condition began clearing. He used oils to help control the stress, and this helped break the vicious circle in which he had been trapped for so long.

Essential oils

Camomile to reduce inflammation. Geranium and lavender are balancing, calming, good for the dry type of eczema. Bergamot and juniper are antiseptic, astringent, and good for the "weeping" type (don't use directly on the skin, use very dilute in bath). Benzoin soothes areas raw from scratching. Myrrh is very healing, good for "weeping" type of eczema. Detoxifying oils and diet can also be a help. Some people swear by evening primrose oil.

These oils can be blended in a simple lotion. I don't usually use carrier oils on eczema, except for calendula. The oils can also be used in cold compresses, or in the bath. Please do a patch test before using them over an extensive area, and make sure you find out about any allergies before you use anything. I would avoid using oils which are related to anything to which the person may be allergic. You should also look at the underlying emotional problems or stress factors that may accompany a particular outbreak, and use oils to help with this, even if only in a burner. The skin may get worse, or very dry and scaly before it gets better, and for people who have been using cortisone or some other quick-acting medication, this may be difficult to accept. This must be understood. There is no quick or easy cure for this condition, although Shirley Price's Problem Skin lotion and Special E Cream hold a reputation for considerably easing the problem.

Recipes for Natural Creams, Toners, and Exfoliants

A basic cleansing lotion

50 cc witch hazel (you can use rose water for dry skin)
10 cc vegetable glycerine
40 cc herbal infusion
a pinch of borax

Dissolve the borax in the herbal infusion and mix with the other ingredients. Add a few drops of essential oil if desired. Keep in a capped bottle in the refrigerator.

A good basic carrier cream

Its texture is heavier than creams bought in the store, but it does liquefy on contact with the skin.

3 tsp beeswax
3 tsp emulsifying wax
½ cup almond oil
½ cup avocado or jojoba or sunflower oil
3 tablespoons rose water

Heat the waxes in the top of a double boiler, and add the vegetable oils. Heat the rose water separately and add a drop at a time to the oil, stirring constantly. Remove from the heat and stir occasionally until cool. Add essential oils as desired.

Cleansing cream (Galen's recipe)

1 ½ tbsp beeswax
1 tbsp emulsifying wax
4 tbsp almond oil
6 tbsp rose water
½ tsp borax
essential oil of rose (or any other you choose)

Heat the rose water with the borax so the borax dissolves. Melt the waxes and oils together in a double boiler. When they are thoroughly melted and mixed, remove both containers from the heat and add the rose water slowly, stirring continuously until the mixture is cool. Then add the essential oil and pour into a jar, keep cool.

Herbal Infusions to Use as Simple Toners

Marigold (calendula) for sensitive skins, elderflower for dry skin, linden flowers for aging skin and wrinkles, yarrow for oily skin. Add one tablespoon of herb to ½ pint of boiling water and allow to cool for an hour. Strain and bottle. Keep refrigerated.

Lavender/bergamot toner for greasy skin and acne

100 cc witch hazel

200 cc orange flower water

3 tsp vodka (to dissolve the oils)

3 drops each of bergamot and lavender oils

Add the essential oils to the vodka before adding to the water and witch hazel. Shake well before use.

You can make toners for other skin types by adding 6 drops of the appropriate essential oils to 3 tsp of vodka and ½ pint of rose water or distilled water.

Exfoliants

Make a mixture of:

⅓ cup ground almonds

⅓ cup ground oatmeal

⅓ cup fine cornmeal or bran

2–3 drops lemon

Put in a clean jar. Moisten a small amount in the palm of your hand, rub into the skin, and rinse well.

You might like to start collecting jars, ingredients, and recipes for natural cosmetics. By trying the different recipes, you can eventually end up with a nice range of your own for all skin types. I can guarantee, if you get used to the textures, that these creams and toners will do far more for your skin than anything on the commercial market, and you will find people asking you for them. Putting them in nice jars and designing a nice label will make them that much more pleasant to use. Try to take creams out of jars with a spatula, and use toners on damp cotton squares. Apply masks with a large brush, and remove with hot towels or washcloths. You can also use a natural sponge. Remember that these cosmetics do not have preservatives, so they have a short shelf life. Make small batches, and keep them refrigerated.

Please do not be taken in by the expensive aromatherapy skin care products on the market. You don't need them, and every experienced aromatherapist I know ends up using their own simple blends of essential oils. They are far more effective and alive than anything you can buy. If you are doing skin treatments for other people, who can resist a blend made especially for them? When I had my clinic, I found that people loved personalized, natural facials, and were far more pleased with their own little brown bottle of custom-blended oil than any expensive commercial product that I could have offered them.

Embrocation

In the tradition of holistic aromatherapy which we are studying, massage is the main method of applying the essential oils. This is not true for all schools of thought in aromatherapy: the French medical tradition, the chemical study of the oils, perfumery, or the spiritual/meditative tradition.

The hands-on application of essential oils, the reliance on their cutaneous absorption, and the particular techniques of aromatherapy massage all began with Madame Maury. She was uncomfortable with the oral administration of essences, and finding that inhalation of the oil had limited and short-term effects, she set out to find a new way. She wrote:

> What we wanted was rejuvenation, the regeneration of the individual. We were looking for an effective way that would be completely harmless. We had to find a method

capable both of influencing the muscular tonus, the quality and aspect of the skin and the tissues, and to obtain a better functioning and a normalization of the individual's rhythm…If we could make the odoriferous matter penetrate direct through the skin into the extra-cellular spaces, and thus into the organic liquids in which the cells bathe; if we could diffuse this fluid matter within a reasonable time and at a reasonable rhythm it would be possible to establish a new treatment and find a new way.[1]

This is exactly what she succeeded in doing. Later she went to England and began teaching. Her massage technique has become the standard taught in aromatherapy courses throughout the world. This is the basic form taught by such English teachers as Patricia Davis, Shirley Price, and Madame Arcier, who was directly trained by Madame Maury.

The aromatherapy massage is a very gentle technique incorporating elements of Swedish massage, polarity, lymphatic work, acupressure, reflexology, and working with subtle energies. Very deep work, or the more vigorous Swedish strokes, are too stimulating when used with the essential oils. When you have a deep understanding of aromatherapy, you can begin to use the oils with a variety of therapeutic techniques. However, Robert Tisserand[2] made a good point when he wrote, "The right essential oils and the wrong massage, or the right massage and the wrong essential oils, will not give positive results."

I've discovered that many of my students who are massage therapists have simply incorporated essential oils into the style of work they already do. I always insist that they carefully consider the type of massage they are doing, and its purposes.

Adding essential oils, which generally increase the circulation, to body work which is very deep or substantially increases circulation, can simply be too stimulating to the body. We cannot forget that in an aromatherapy massage, the oils are doing a great deal of the therapeutic work. They are not added merely for a pleasant scent.

Thus it is not enough to apply the essential oils haphazardly; a true understanding of the oils, knowledge of their effects on the body, and the aims of aromatherapy treatment all are necessary. Some of you reading this book may be massage therapists, or have some training in massage. If you have no experience, at some point you will need to get some practical training, because this approach to aromatherapy centers on the use of massage in treatment.

Diagnostic techniques used with aromatherapy include reflexology, iridology, and muscle testing. Some practitioners also employ dowsing, and if they are trained in herbalism, homeopathy, or oriental medicine, they use various other traditional skills such as tongue or urine analysis. We must always remember that we are not physicians, and cannot diagnose or prescribe.

Effects and Benefits of Massage

Combining the essential oils with massage gives us double benefit: the healing power of touch and massage and the plant energy of the essential oils. In this section we will discuss the benefits of massage, and in the next will examine how the oils penetrate the skin and influence the body from inside.

Two of the most obvious benefits of massage are the healing power of touch and the exchange of energy that takes place between therapist and client. We know that touch is a basic need, and that babies who are not handled become sick and die. Unfortunately, in our culture smell and touch are lost senses, although the value of massage was recognized in ancient Greece. The word itself is a Greek work meaning "to knead," and Hippocrates said, "..it is necessary to rub the shoulder gently and smoothly with soft hands. The physician must be experienced in many things, but assuredly also in rubbing." Some well-known physical benefits of massage are:

- Increasing circulation to the tissues of the body. This brings fresh blood and nutrients, and carries away waste products. The essential oils are also transported by the bloodstream to the areas in the body where they are needed. Massage towards the heart will assist in venous flow.

- Loosening of tight muscles. They can be tight because of lack of use, or too much use, and massage using techniques and oils chosen to work specifically on the muscles can help with this. It is also true that very often the muscles hold emotions that we have stored there, and massage, the reassurance of a therapist's touch, and a sensitive choice and use of oils aimed at working on this level can go a long way towards helping the release and balancing of these emotions. Rose and geranium would be a good combination for emotional balance. Using this oil with various techniques, plus work on the heart chakra, has led to some very powerful emotional releases. Men who are afraid to show their emotions are often very surprised at the power of the rose. A blend of marjoram, lavender, rosemary, and a drop of ginger is good for relaxing and warming the muscles.

- Cleansing the system and releasing of toxins. For the oils to be efficiently absorbed by the body, the skin and tissues should be as free of toxins and congestion as possible. Some practitioners request that all of their clients go on a cleansing regime before commencing serious treatment with the oils. Blends can also be created that will help with purification and detoxification of the body. Juniper, rosemary, and lemon is a good blend for this. I've often been told by clients that after using such a blend, the room they visit most frequently during the next 24 hours is the bathroom. Sometimes they even have to go during the massage! I encourage them to drink as much water as possible after their treatment.

- Relieving pain in a particular area. Analgesic oils such as marjoram and lavender will help with this. We know that natural painkillers such as endorphins are released through acupuncture, they may also be released through massage.

- Enhancing lymphatic flow in the body. Specific massage techniques have been developed to work on the lymphatic system. Excess fluid can be controlled, and thus we can relieve stress on the kidneys and other organs of elimination. Diuretic oils such as geranium can be added to the massage oil to make our lymphatic work more effective. We also know that the immune system relies on the lymphatic system for its efficient functioning. Since the lymphatic system has no pump, it relies on muscular movement for efficient flow. Many people with sedentary life styles have very sluggish immune systems, and regular massage can be of great help in making immune functioning more efficient. This can be enhanced in aromatherapy massage by using immunity enhancing oils such as tea-tree and eucalyptus.

• Making the client more aware of his or her body. Grounding oils such as patchouli, sandalwood, and vetivert are helpful if you believe that this is an appropriate level on which to work. Alternatively, you can use grounding oils on the feet. Sometimes specific areas seem "dead"; for example, a very cold lower back. Warming oils such as ginger, rosemary, and black pepper can be used in dilute form on these specific areas.

More and more massage therapists work on the energetic systems of the body, as in working with the meridian system, the chakras, or other elements such as the aura. Although these are non-physical, we can apply oils in a vibrational way, and they can be used with crystal, color, sound, etc.

For many people massage is an important way to relax and deal with stress, and we know it facilitates the release of certain neurochemical substances and a general relaxation of the nervous system. The techniques used in aromatherapy massage are designed to be relaxing rather than stimulating, and wonderful sedative blends containing oils which specifically relax the nervous system, such as lavender, sandalwood, and clary sage can be created.

Massage always entails the sharing of energies between two people. If the therapist is in tune, this happens on the emotional as well as the physical level. When essential oils are used, the therapist is influenced by them too; this creates a further bond between the two parties. You will often find that the clients you attract at a particular time will echo issues you are working on in your own life. When working with oils, you must allow half an hour between clients, if you are not to be totally spaced out by the end of your working day!

I especially remember a busy day when I didn't follow this rule, and during my last massage I broke into uncontrollable laughter. My client began laughing too, and we had to abandon the session and reschedule it for the next day. Recalling the old saying that laughter is the best medicine, maybe that is just what she needed!

We should also remember that by working on certain areas of the body, such as the hands and feet in reflexology, intense and careful work along the spine, using the dermatomes, and working along the main meridians, we are indirectly affecting the organs and major body systems. Aromatherapy massage incorporates this type of work. Oils which correspond to specific organs or body systems can be used on specific zones or meridians to enhance the effect of massage. For example, rosemary and rose could be used on the liver area of the foot in a reflexology treatment. Many clients feel the energy moving from the area of the foot to the corresponding area of the body. This seems to take the form of a little twinge or even a burst of energy moving up the reflex zone.

Finally, we must consider the benefits of self-nurturing and self-massage for the therapist. Giving a good massage to someone else depends on being clear, centered, balanced and nurtured yourself. All aromatherapists must take time to treat themselves, and that includes living and working with the oils on a daily basis.

Contraindications of Massage

Despite all of the wonderful benefits listed, do not massage someone who has had recent surgery, has cancer, is undergoing chemotherapy, has a fever or infection, has a history of thrombosis, broken bones that have not healed completely, severe burns, skin disorders, or extreme acne. If your client is pregnant, do not massage the stomach. Also check for any contraindications to the use of certain oils.

How Can Cutaneous Application Be Effective?

Many people will ask how applying the oils in a massage can do any good. Surely the best way is to swallow them? Let's look in more detail at how they penetrate the skin and enter the bloodstream.

The skin is the body's largest organ, and is one of the most important organs of elimination. The state of our skin tells a great deal about the state of our body: if toxins and waste products are being eliminated efficiently, if the fluid balance is correct, if our glands are functioning efficiently, how well we are processing the nourishment we take in, how well our circulation is working, our mental and emotional state, and so on. Before we begin working with the oils, a quick examination of the skin will give us a good idea about the state of the body's systems. As was mentioned earlier, applying the oils to a very congested skin is much less effective therapeutically, and absorption by the body is much slower. This is also the case for very obese people.

If you intend using the oils therapeutically on a client, and you see indications of body toxicity, suggest a fruit diet for two or three days before the massage. Explain that this will enable the body to utilize the oils more efficiently and effectively.

I have noticed that as people use the oils over a long period of time they become much more sensitive to them, and it takes far less essential oil to achieve a desired result. This is probably because their body systems are much cleaner, more balanced, and more efficient after using the oils regularly.

Another function of the skin is to serve as a protective outer covering, and this is important if harmful substances are to be kept out. However, the skin is semipermeable, which means that certain substances of small molecular size can pass through. Substances such as lanolin have large molecules and sit on the skin, acting as a barrier. This makes lanolin good as a protective cream, but of no use in aromatherapy when we want the essential oils to penetrate. Vegetable oils such as grapeseed, almond, sunflower, and jojoba (a vegetable wax) are much better carrier oils.

Essential oil molecules are small enough to penetrate the skin, and this enables us to use them externally to achieve internal effects. They also dissolve in oil, so the sebum of the skin helps to dissolve them even further, making it easier for them to penetrate. Applying a mild source of heat or manual friction to the area will help to open the pores and increase the circulation. However, when the skin is perspiring heavily, such as after a sauna, it will not absorb.

When we have diluted the essential oil in a carrier oil and applied it to a fairly porous skin, the oil molecules are absorbed and pass into the fluid which surrounds every cell. From there they pass through the thin walls of the capillaries and small lymph ducts which lie below the surface. Thus the circulatory and lymphatic systems pick up the oils and carry them throughout the body. It is estimated that it takes about ten to twenty minutes for the oils to get into the blood stream, but up to three to six hours for them to be completely absorbed by the body, any surplus passes out in the urine after two to eight hours. For this reason, it is best not to bathe or shower for three to six hours after an aromatherapy massage, so please ask your clients to shower before applying the oils.

Madame Maury wrote of the absorption of essential oils through the skin:

> It was possible, therefore, to reach this extra-cellular liquid (it represents 27 percent if the mass of our body, without counting other biological liquids), and it could be acted upon through a healthy and receptive skin. This diffusion takes place by exchanges between the extra-cellular and lacunary liquids and the blood, the lymph and the tissues. The elements introduced are carried by the liquids to the organs and retained selectively by the latter. [3]

In verification of the last sentence of the quote above, mice were injected with rosemary, and when they were dissected, a large concentration of rosemary oil was found in the liver, as expected. Rose seems to target the uterus, camomile the digestive system, rosemary and lavender the nervous system. As you study, take note of the specific affinity of certain oils for certain areas of the body. In my classes

I often have students smell an oil and try to tune into the part of the body it affects. Nine times out of ten they correctly identify the organ or body system for which the oil has an affinity.

When oils are applied in the correct quantities, the body will accept what it needs and reject the excess, which will be excreted via the breath, perspiration, urine, or feces. Different oils will be eliminated through different routes; the greater part of garlic oil is eliminated through the lungs, while sandalwood is eliminated through the urine. If an oil is misused, it can cause poisoning and irreversibly damage the liver or some other organ so much that fatality results.

Many people advocate oral use of the oils, particularly the French physicians who prescribe them in capsules. The operative word here is physicians. Both British independent associations totally discourage internal use, and there are studies which show damage of the stomach lining by essential oils when taken incorrectly or in excessive amounts. Furthermore, unless you are a physician, it is unlawful for you to prescribe oils in this way.

Applying the oils to the skin is also a far more efficient way to get oils into the body. In an emergency, massaging someone every 15 minutes or so would enable you to get a much larger quantity of oils into the body than would be tolerable by mouth. In a normal dosage, both systems deliver about the same quantity of essential oils into the system: three drops.

Making Your Basic Massage Oil

The usual ratio of essential oil to carrier in massage oils is between one and a half to three percent. This means you add nine to eighteen drops of essential oil to each ounce of carrier oil. If you want to make a smaller quantity, you can add three drops of essential oil to one teaspoon of carrier oil.

The carrier oils I like best for general massage are rice bran, safflower, grapeseed, or jojoba oil, although jojoba has become very expensive. If I want to make my basic oil richer, I add up to ten percent of avocado, which aids penetration, wheatgerm, which adds vitamin E and helps prevent oxidation, or almond oil, a nice oil for facial massage.

Here are some recipes for massage oil that I find particularly useful, although you know that as a professional aromatherapist you will be creating individual blends for your clients.

Muscular aches and pains and sports massage: lavender, clary sage, marjoram, lemon, ginger, black pepper, rosemary.

Joints: lemon, rosemary, marjoram, juniper.

Detoxification: juniper, lemon, geranium, rosemary, cypress.

Lymphatic work: cypress, juniper, geranium, rosemary, tea-tree, eucalyptus, lemon, thyme for immune enhancement.

Emotionally calming: rose, geranium, lavender, neroli, ylang-ylang, sandalwood, camomile.

Sedative massage: lavender, clary sage, marjoram, ylang-ylang, sandalwood, neroli, vetivert.

Stimulating: peppermint (in small quantities), rosemary, juniper, basil, black pepper, ginger, cinnamon, lemon.

Aphrodisiac: vetivert, sandalwood, patchouli, ylang-ylang, rose, jasmine, cinnamon, ginger, clary sage.

There are many blended massage oils on the market, and these are fine to start with. However, I encourage you to experiment with creating blends of your own, and once you are working with clients, always to blend individually wherever possible. This is the heart and soul of aromatherapy practice.

In concluding this chapter, I suggest that you obtain Shirley Price's book.[4] It contains a detailed explanation of an aromatherapy massage, with diagrams to guide you. While not a complete training in aromatherapy massage, it will give you something to start working with.

Endnotes

1. Maury, M. *Marguerite Maury's Guide to Aromatherapy: The Secret of Life and Youth.* Saffron Walden, England: C. W. Daniel, 1989.

2. Tisserand, R. *The Art of Aromatherapy.* Saffron Walden, England: C. W. Daniel, 1977.

3. Maury, M. *Marguerite Maury's Guide to Aromatherapy: The Secret of Life and Youth.* Saffron Walden, England: C. W. Daniel, 1989.

4. Price, S. *Practical Aromatherapy: How to Use Essential Oils to Restore Vitality.* Wellingborough, England: Thorsons, 1987.

9

The Second Circulatory System

The lymphatic system is one of the most interesting body systems, and is one that aromatherapists can work with directly and effectively. In this chapter we will look at the structure and function of this "second circulatory system" and how we can work to increase its efficiency by using essential oils and specific massage techniques.

Structure of the Lymphatic System

The lymphatic system comprises a network of superficial and deep vessels which are found in all parts of the body except the brain and spinal column and areas such as bone marrow and cartilage that receive nutrition through diffusion rather than from blood vessels.

The two main structures of this system are the lymph capillaries, vessels and larger ducts, which make up the network for the transport of lymph, and the lymph nodes, which are the filtering devices. Valves in the network of vessels control the flow of lymph and direct it towards the main drainage areas, the right and left subclavian veins. It is here that the lymph rejoins the bloodstream via the thoracic and right lymph ducts.

The left side of the body, the lower limbs, pelvis, perineum, abdominal viscera, left thorax, left arm, left side of the head and neck drain into the thoracic duct and the left subclavian vein. The right half of the thorax, right arm, right side of the head and neck drain into the right lymph duct, and into the right subclavian vein. About three fourths of the toxins circulating in the lymph are found on the left side of the body; good drainage is necessary for elimination of these toxins.

Unlike the circulatory system, the lymphatic system has no pump, and relies on muscular compression and general body activity for moving the lymphatic fluid around the body. This is why lack of exercise, poor muscle tone, sedentary work, and jobs which require excessive standing can lead to edema and an inefficient immune system. It is also why massage can be an effective treatment for a sluggish lymphatic system.

The lymph nodes are the filtering sites for the lymphatic fluid, which is a transparent, watery fluid resembling blood plasma but containing less protein and more lymphocytes. These are composed of lymphoid tissue, and are found singly or in groups near veins. They range in size from a pinhead to an olive, but are generally about the size of a kidney bean.

There are about 600 to 700 lymph nodes throughout the body; those most easily felt on the body surface are the cervical nodes (under the mandible and in front of the ear), the axillary nodes (under the arm), and the inguinal nodes (in the groin). There are also nodes in the popliteal fossa (behind the knee), occipital area (base of the skull), and the cupital area (at the elbow).

The spleen, thymus, and tonsils are considered lymphatic organs, and the breast is largely made up of lymphatic glands and vessels.

Functions of the Lymphatic System

The lymphatic system serves three main functions in the body:

Absorption and distribution of fat-soluble nutrients

In the small intestine, small lymphatic vessels are in contact with the intestinal wall. The villi, which are minute projections on the wall, enclose lacteal ducts which are also in contact with the small lymphatic vessels. Blood capillaries are also found in the villi. Sugars,

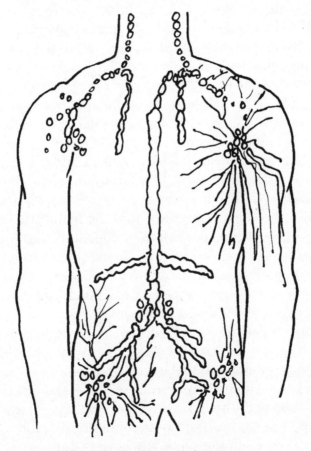

The Lymphatic System

minerals, amino acids, water-soluble vitamins and a few fatty substances are absorbed into the bloodstream via these capillaries. Fatty nutrients and the fat-soluble vitamins are absorbed into the lymphatic system via the lacteals. Directly (via the hepatic portal system of the circulatory system), or indirectly (via the lymphatic system), these nutrients are carried to the liver, where the fat-soluble vitamins are stored. They are also carried to the cells as nourishment. There are also small lymph nodes in the small intestine which provide antibodies against microorganisms that may find their way there.

Drainage of excess fluid from body cells and tissues

One of the main functions of the lymphatic system is to control the volume of fluid circulating in the body. Interstitial fluid is composed of blood plasma (the transparent, watery part of the blood), which filters through the thin walls of the capillaries into the surrounding connective tissues. Most of the proteins in the plasma remain in the blood, and this helps to draw some of the fluid back into the capillaries by osmosis. The interstitial fluid is vital to the cells. It brings moisture and nutrients, and picks up the waste products of cell metabolism, excess proteins, bacteria, viruses, and inorganic material such as dyes and chemicals, to be transported to the organs of elimination. Not all fluid is drawn back into the capillaries, and this becomes lymph, which is absorbed into the lymphatic vessels and carried away to the lymph nodes for filtering, thus cleansing the fluid before it returns to the bloodstream via the subclavian veins. Poor lymphatic drainage results in excessive fluid in the tissues, which causes edema and a strain on the kidneys, heart, and other avenues of fluid excretion. Pronounced edema may in fact be a sign of heart or kidney damage or disease and should not be neglected.

Thus, the body contains two circulatory systems: blood and lymph; both carry nutrients to the cells, both remove waste products from the cells, and both are concerned with maintaining the level of fluid circulating in the body. Because the lymphatic system does not have a pump like the heart, it can become sluggish and inefficient, particularly if we get little exercise and have a poor diet, which loads cells with waste products that are difficult to eliminate.

Fighting infection

The lymphatic system helps fight infection in two ways:

1. Lymph nodes manufacture lymphocytes, which make up 23 percent of the white blood cells. Lymphocytes in turn manufacture antibodies, which are complex proteins with the capacity to neutralize antigens or invading bacteria. The enlargement of lymph nodes indicates the production of large numbers of lymphocytes when an infection is present, or when the body is on the defensive. Granulocytes, which are white blood cells made in the bone marrow, also help in this process, and ingest foreign bacteria in a process known as phagocytosis. They migrate out of the capillaries and accumulate around areas of infection to engulf the invading microbes. The rise in the general metabolic rate which produces a fever during infectious illnesses is due to the increased production of antibodies and white blood cells. Lymphocytes and antibodies are also produced in the spleen and thymus glands. The spleen also filters lymph like a large lymph node, and contains considerable lymphoid tissue.

2. Lymph nodes also are the filtering stations for the lymphatic system. They comprise a network of fibers in which are found white blood cells called macrophages which ingest foreign bodies as the lymph passes through the nodes.

Methods of Assessing Poor Lymphatic Performance

One of the main indicators of a sluggish lymphatic system is edema (swelling) of the face or body. We all have seen swollen ankles on people who are on their feet all day. Pregnancy, with its increased weight, extra volume of blood and fluid and hormonal changes, can be accompanied by edema. Walking and elevating the legs can help relieve the condition.

Temporary edema can occur around injuries such as a sprained ankle, when damage to the tissues can interfere with the exchange and drainage of fluids. Cold compresses and ice packs can help reduce swelling, and massage from above the site of the injury towards the lymph glands can help start the fluid moving.

PMS (premenstrual syndrome) can be a time of insufficient fluid elimination, when hormones can influence the efficiency of fluid exchange and elimination. Lymphatic massage, which we will discuss later, can considerably reduce this problem over time.

Persistent edema can be symptomatic of something more serious, such as heart or kidney disease, and if treatment produces no improvement, a physician must be consulted.

Fluid imbalances can also lead to mineral imbalances in the body that could be dangerous, and the extended use of diuretics, even mild natural ones, is not recommended.

Puffiness in the face can also be a sign of insufficient lymphatic drainage. Massaging in the direction of the lymph nodes can help to reduce this. Spongy tissue on the body is also a sign that fluids are not being removed effectively.

Cellulite can be another consequence of poor lymphatic drainage. This is characterized by spongy, often painful areas on the thighs and buttocks, and sometimes on the arms. A good way to recognize cellulite is to form the thumbs and forefingers of the hands into a diamond shape, and to squeeze the area in question. If cellulite is present, the area will take on a dimpled, pitted appearance. The skin may also retain the indentation of your fingers, and it may feel cold, grainy, and lumpy. Ordinary fat will not do this. There are many causes of cellulite, and most women probably will suffer from it at some time during their life. Some physicians link it to a hormonal imbalance, and others specifically attribute it to excess estrogen, which may explain why it is more common among women than men. Men who drink beer excessively sometimes have it, possibly due to the plant estrogen in the beer.

Cellulite can also be caused by poor circulation and poor lymphatic drainage, which means that excess toxins and fluid accumulate in the tissues. Some researchers link it with allergies and imbalances in the endocrine system.

Over time, a sluggish lymphatic system and poor local circulation, plus a high level of toxins in the body, can mean that gradually a whole area of the body becomes stagnant. Eventually, physical changes occur in the cells. The capillaries become stretched and walls weaken. Blood plasma leaks out into the fatty layer, and the spaces between fat cells become filled with fluid. This causes bumpiness and tenderness if nerve endings become compressed. The walls of the fat cells also become thickened by a layer of connective tissue, and this makes the process of fluid exchange even more difficult.

In my practice, I've found that most women have some degree of edema or cellulite. With men, there is often some degree of lymphatic congestion, usually due to poor living habits or stress. I usually include some lymphatic work with every client, and I'd go so far as to say that if I had to choose only one form of massage therapy for people without specific injuries, lymphatic massage would be it.

Of course, essential oils add an entirely new dimension to manual lymph drainage techniques. Many of my students and fellow aromatherapists report that an added bonus to their work with the oils is a much stronger immune system, and I can attest to this.

How Aromatherapy Can Help Lymphatic Problems

We aromatherapists can help overcome some problems in the lymphatic system by using carefully selected essential oils that have a particular affinity with the processes involved. The oils we choose when working with the lymphatic system will have these characteristics: they will be diuretic, circulatory stimulants, hormonal balancers, oils which increase leucocytosis, blood cleansers and detoxifiers, bactericidal oils, antiviral oils, antifungal oils, and oils which help to accelerate lymph and tissue fluid circulation. The effects of essential oils on the immune system have been studied extensively by French researchers and physicians, and this is one of the main applications advocated by medical aromatherapists.

Diuretics: Fennel, grapefruit, cypress, lemon, juniper (be careful, excessive use of juniper has been known to cause kidney damage). These can also be used in the form of herbal infusions.

Circulatory stimulants: Black pepper, rosemary, or ginger. Use sparingly, massaging towards the heart and lymph nodes; you might use one or two drops in a lymphatic massage blend.

Hormonal balancers: Geranium, fennel, rose, cypress, clary sage.

Increase leucocytosis (manufacture of white blood cells): Bergamot, lavender, lemon, camomile, rosemary, thyme, sage.

Blood cleansers, detoxifiers: All essential oils stimulate phagocytosis to some degree. (Phagocytosis is the ability of the white blood cells to gobble up invaders.) Specifically: juniper, lemon (helps eliminate uric acid), camomile (for high urea levels), lemongrass and rosemary (for lactic acid buildup in muscles), garlic (thins and cleanses the blood), rosemary and marjoram (laxatives), eucalyptus, peppermint, tea-tree, and sandalwood (expectorants), rosemary and ginger (sudorifics, which help increase perspiration). All help in the elimination of excess waste products and make the job of the lymphatic system easier.

Bactericidal oils: Camomile, garlic, lavender, lemon, and clove. All essential oils are antiseptic and bactericidal to some degree, with specific oils being more effective with specific microbes. According to Robert Tisserand,[1] tea-tree is specific to streptococcus, gonococcus, and pneumococcus. Sandalwood is specific to staphylococcus aurens, which is present in infected wounds, abscesses, and boils, thyme to e. coli, which is found with some kidney infections, lemon helps with c. diphtheriae, cinnamon with typhus bacillus, and clove with m. tuberculosis. Obviously, aromatherapists will not deal with these diseases, but this list shows how essential oils can help the immune system combat infectious diseases by attacking the microbes.

Antiviral oils: Essential oils can be very useful against viruses, while few drugs can deal with them. Viral infections include colds, herpes, chicken pox, shingles, the various influenzas, and measles. Useful oils are cinnamon, thyme, black pepper, eucalyptus, tea-tree (for some influenza and cold viruses), lavender and melissa (for herpes simplex or cold sores), and geranium (for shingles).

Antifungal oils: Lavender, myrrh, tea-tree (also effective against candida albicans).

Oils which stimulate the lymphatic system: Sage, lavender, and rosemary. Dr. Gumbel[2] suggests peppermint as a key oil for the lymphatic system. He says it accelerates lymph and tissue fluid circulation, and "...has a special connection to everything aqueous, to blood, to tissue fluid, lymph, spinal and cerebral fluid." Peppermint is also used for the care of dried, atrophied skin, since it supports water retention and activates tissue fluid circulation. If used on the face it must be very dilute, and kept well away from the eyes. A peppermint water spray could be effective.

We can also help lymphatic problems by using specific lymphatic drainage massage techniques. If you are not a massage therapist, you can enhance the efficiency of the lymphatic system by simply massaging the oils into the body in the direction of the major lymph nodes, and finally, the subclavian veins. This means that from the feet you would massage upwards towards the groin, and from the midline of the body down. For the axillary nodes, you would massage from the hand upwards, and from the rib area, pectoral area, and shoulder area you would massage downwards to the nodes. From the clavicle you would massage up to the cervical nodes, and from the face would be downwards to the cervical nodes or the right lymphatic duct and thoracic duct on the left-hand side.

The massage should be slow and rhythmic, done in a pumping movement, if possible. Before starting the massage, dry skin brushing is a good idea to stimulate circulation, again in the directions indicated. You could also apply oil directly to the lymph nodes, thymus, kidney and spleen areas.

If you are a reflexology practitioner, applying oils to the lymphatic areas of the feet is a good way to get the oils into the lymphatic system. Adding them to a cream is an easier way to work with them on the feet. You could use either the oils designed to move lymph and fluid, or the oils for the immune system, on these areas in addition to your lymphatic massage work.

In an unpublished lecture, Dr. Penoel suggested skin brushing along the meridian pathway, and deep foot reflexology. He also recommended applying oils to the lymphatic sites, the solar plexus, breasts (remember how much lymph tissue is here), the area of the adrenal glands, the spleen, and liver. Diffusers are also used.

In an acute situation, the French medical aromatherapists will put as much as 15 ml of straight essential oil into the system. This is something best left to physicians, because it is potentially dangerous.

Several methods of lymphatic drainage massage have emerged. The classic aromatherapy massage developed by Maury and Arcier incorporates a lot of lymphatic work. The best-known system of lymphatic massage was developed in the 1930s by Dr. Emil Vodder when he and his wife were working as masseurs at the French Riviera. They noticed that all of their English clients had chronic respiratory problems and swollen lymph nodes. Dr. Vodder developed a system of movements which drained the lymph nodes and relieved the symptoms. He spent the next 40 years developing a system of lymphatic drainage massage which is now taught all over Europe.

Even if you do a simple stroking, pumping massage to move the lymph, you need to be aware of the contraindications to this type of massage, and observe them very rigidly. Manual lymph drainage must not be done on anyone who has active cancer, heart trouble, thrombosis, phlebitis, high blood pressure, varicose veins, pregnancy, any acute inflammation or infection, or any other severe medical problem. This method should not be used on anyone who has undergone recent chemotherapy, since the toxins stored in the blood and liver will be quickly released into the bloodstream and make the person feel very ill.

Professionally qualified practitioners can use this method successfully on patients who have had a mastectomy, when the lymph nodes have been removed and this has produced a build-up of fluid in the arm. I must emphasize again that this must not be attempted by anyone who has not been fully trained in this method.

For cellulite, there are a number of measures that can be taken to help detoxify the area, increase circulation and lymphatic movement, and flush excess fluid from the tissues.

In all work with the lymphatic system, diet is important, because a highly refined diet full of chemicals and potential toxic by-products makes the job of waste removal much harder for the system. Anyone serious about improving lymphatic and immune function must stop smoking and eliminate junk food, red meat, coffee, tea, alcohol, refined white sugar, flour and milk products from their diet. In fact, a three-day fruit fast is a good way to start. Herbal infusions such as fennel should be consumed, and at least eight glasses of water a day will help to flush the system.

Regular massage, ideally every day but at least twice a week, is important to help improve the circulation of blood and lymph and break down and disperse the toxic deposits in the tissues. This would incorporate the appropriate essential oils in a cream, because oils make the skin too slippery.

An exercise program is important, and gentle, rhythmic walking or swimming is appropriate for the cellulite problem. Baths can be useful, and brisk friction over the area before entering the bath is helpful. This can be done with a loofah or body brush. While in the bath, pinch and pummel the area to help break down fatty deposits.

Adding Epsom salts, sea salt, or seaweed extracts to the bath can also help eliminate toxins, and this should be done twice a week. After the bath, apply a cellulite blend over the areas you are treating and rub in well. Skin brushing, bathing in oils, and massage with the cellulite blend should be done once a day.

The best oils for cellulite are juniper, grapefruit, lemon, cypress, fennel, thyme, rosemary, basil, and patchouli. You can also use the diuretic oils, and occasionally add a drop of black pepper to help increase the circulation to the area. Geranium will help to balance hormones. On the following page are three anticellulite massage formulas.

Use 15 to 20 drops of essential oil in one ounce of carrier oil. The best carrier oils are almond oil, jojoba, or carrot.

1. Juniper   8 drops
   Lemon   5 drops
   Rosemary   5 drops

2. Geranium   7 drops
   Rosemary   6 drops
   Basil   4 drops

3. Grapefruit   6 drops
   Lemon   5 drops
   Juniper   4 drops

Much of my work with women in a salon setting has been on skin care and cellulite treatments. Provided that the client has been motivated to follow the complete program of diet, exercise, and aromatherapy, I've seen spectacular results from using specific massage techniques and appropriate essential oils.

One woman told me that she saw great results after only two treatments and using the oil blend for a few weeks. This won't happen to everyone, but it can be an effective regimen for women who haven't been able to do anything with their "thunder thighs." An added benefit is their increased self-esteem and self-confidence.

Remember that anything that helps the lymphatic system also will help the immune system, and you could devise a similar routine of detoxifying baths, skin brushing, and massage using slow, rhythmic movements towards the direction of the lymph nodes, using the appropriate immune-enhancing oils. Tea-tree, eucalyptus, lemon, thyme, or rosemary would be especially appropriate.

Endnotes

1. Tisserand, R. *To Heal and Tend the Body.* Wilmot, Wisconsin: Lotus Press, 1988.

2. Gumbel, G. *Principles of Holistic Skin Therapy with Herbal Essences.* Heidelberg, Germany: Haug, 1986.

10

The Body's Regulators

The endocrine system is one of the most interesting and beautifully tuned body systems. Working with the nervous system, it is an agent of homeostasis, coordinating many body processes and activities, so when it is out of balance we feel it emotionally, mentally, and physically. Body processes regulated by the endocrine system include: promotion and inhibition of organ functions, growth, reproductive cycles and activity, and balancing of the body's metabolism.

In this chapter we will discuss the structure and functions of the system, the hormones produced by it, and the organs they affect. We will also consider the link between olfaction and the endocrine system, which is very important for aromatherapists. Various chakras have been linked traditionally with the endocrine glands, and this will be discussed, as well as the direct and indirect effects that essential oils can have on hormonal balance.

We will also look at why some essential oils work as aphrodisiacs, and how we can use them to enhance our sexuality. Finally, for those interested in reflexology, we will look at the areas of the feet which correspond to the main endocrine glands.

The Structure and Function of the Endocrine System

The organs of the endocrine system are the endocrine, or ductless glands. They are called ductless because they secrete their hormones directly into the bloodstream via the capillaries surrounding them, or into the interstitial fluids. The hormones secreted are like chemical messengers, influencing organs and parts of the body a long way from the site of the gland as they travel through the bloodstream. The word hormone is derived from the Greek "to excite," although some hormones stimulate a particular activity and others inhibit it. When a hormone acts as an inhibitory agent it is called a chalone.

There are also exocrine glands in the body, which secrete hormones, enzymes, and other substances into cavities or ducts; the effect of the material secreted is local, because it does not enter the bloodstream. Examples of exocrine glands are the sebaceous and mammary glands, the sweat glands, and the salivary glands.

Small areas of endocrine tissue are also found in the pancreas, testes, ovaries, gastro-intestinal system, and the placenta sometimes secretes hormones.

The Pineal Gland

The pineal gland is a reddish-gray body the size of a pea and the shape of a pine cone. For a long time the pineal was considered a vestigial organ without much use. Recent research indicates that it has something to do with the circadian rhythms of our bodies. There also is evidence that it exerts an inhibitory influence on testicular and ovarian activity through secretion of the hormone melatonin, which appears to affect the central nervous system in response to changes in environmental light. Descartes considered the pineal gland to be the seat of the soul. It has links to the hypothalamus through nervous pathways.

The Hypothalamus and the Pituitary Gland

The hypothalamus, which is actually part of the brain situated in the forebrain, acts as an interface between the nervous system and the endocrine system. It is involved with regulation of the autonomic nervous system, pituitary secretions, integration of autonomic and emotional reactions, appetite, and regulation of body temperature.

Directly beneath and attached to the hypothalamus is the pituitary gland. It is linked to the hypothalamus by portal vessels and secretory neurons; hormones released by the hypothalamus directly influence hormonal secretion by the pituitary. Together, they control and regulate a number of metabolic functions as well as the activity of other endocrine glands.

The pituitary gland is a reddish-gray vascular mass, oval in shape, 1.2 by 1.5 cm in size, located at the base of the skull about two inches behind a point between the eyebrows, and has two lobes, the anterior (adenohypophysis) and posterior (neurohypophysis).

Secretions from the hypothalamus stimulate the anterior lobe of the pituitary to produce seven important hormones:

TSH: Thyroid stimulating hormone or thyrotropin. This stimulates the thyroid gland to produce thyroxine.

FSH: Follicle stimulating hormone. This stimulates the Graafian follicles in the ovary to produce estrogen, and the *corpora lutea* to secrete progesterone in the female; in the male it stimulates the production of testosterone and sperm in the testes.

ACTH: Adrenal cortex stimulating hormone or adrenocorticotrophic hormone. This stimulates the adrenal cortex to produce hormones such as cortisone.

LH: Luteinizing hormone which stimulates the ovaries and testes to

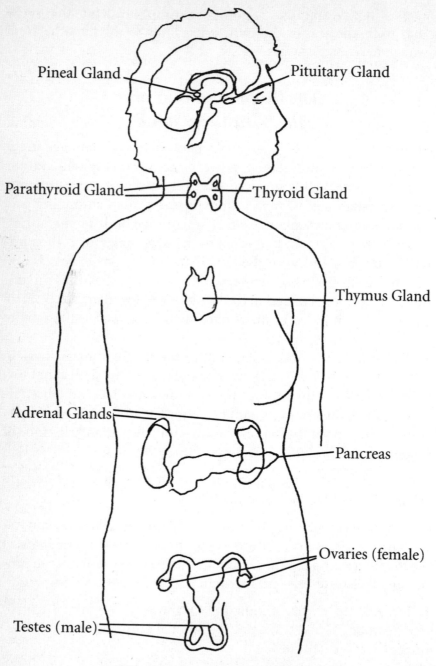

The Endocrine System

release sex hormones, and stimulates the ovaries to produce a *corpus luteum.*

STH: Somatropin, or growth hormone. This stimulates growth, especially of the long bones. Stunted growth or excessive height are due to imbalances of this hormone.

MSH: Melanocyte stimulating hormone. This controls pigmentation in the skin.

Prolactin: Stimulates the mammary glands to produce milk.

The posterior lobe of the pituitary gland has no secretory cells of its own. Hormones from the hypothalamus are secreted by secretory neurons which extend into the posterior lobe. They are oxytocin, which stimulates the release of milk and contraction of the uterus during labor, and ADH, antidiuretic hormone, which controls the concentration of urine by increasing the amount of water reabsorbed by kidney tubules.

The Thyroid and Parathyroid Glands

The thyroid gland weighs about 30 grams and lies just below the larynx or voice box in the neck. It consists of two lobes, right and left, and the four parathyroid glands are located on the posterior side.

The thyroid hormone thyroxine is released in response to the TSH released by the pituitary gland. Thyroxine maintains the metabolic rate by regulating oxygen consumption by the tissues. Oxygen is the prime fuel for metabolic activity in the body and cell respiration. In children, thyroxine is necessary for normal growth, and a deficiency can result in dwarfism and mental retardation. In adults, deficiency can manifest itself as slowness, listlessness, coldness, puffiness, and obesity. Another manifestation of thyroid imbalance is goiter—the swelling of the actual gland.

Iodine helps the production of thyroxine, which is why it is necessary in the diet. Excessive thyroxine secretion results in weight loss, nervousness, tremors, rapid metabolic rate, and protruding eyeballs.

The parathyroid glands regulate the level of calcium in the blood by means of the hormone parathormone, which regulates calcium level by releasing it from bone tissue. Vitamin D is also crucial to calcium homeostasis. Cardiac and other muscular activity relies on adequate calcium levels, as does blood clotting. Insufficient parathyroid functioning produces muscle cramps, stiffness, and spasms. Too much parathormone leads to excessive calcium levels in the blood, producing decalcification of the bones, kidney stones, and calcium deposits.

The Thymus Gland

The thymus gland is located between the thyroid gland and the heart. It consists of two lateral lobes held together by connective tissue, and is encapsulated. It is five cm in length and about five cm in width, but decreases in size after puberty under the influence of the sex hormones, and is almost nonexistent in old age, as the immune system of the body diminishes.

The thymus is linked closely to the immune system, and produces a hormone, thymosin, promoting the development of T-lymphocytes, which boost cellular immunity and are important in the production of antibodies called interferon (antiviral) and lysozym. The thymus is also thought to have a strengthening effect on other lymphatic organs such as the spleen, tonsils, and lymph nodes. There is some evidence that it is influenced by the pituitary.

The Adrenal or Supradrenal Glands

The adrenals lie just above the kidneys like two little hats. They comprise an outer layer, the cortex, and an inner layer, the medulla. The cortex makes up 80 percent of the adrenal and the medulla the rest. The parts really function as two different glands.

The adrenal cortex, made up of the outer layer of the glands, produces a number of different hormones. It secretes aldosterone and other mineralocorticoids which deal with the fluid and electrolyte balances in the body; hormones dealing with carbohydrate metabolism such as cortisol and other glucocoticoids, and low levels of sex hormones, called androcorticoids. Some estrogen is produced here, and this becomes important when none is being produced by the ovaries after menopause.

The medulla releases two hormones, epinephrine (adrenaline) and noradrenaline, which are released in response to fear, stress, or anxiety. This is called the "fight or flight" response, in which increased blood supply is sent to the muscles, blood is rerouted from the skin and the gastrointestinal tract, the heart and respiration rates speed up, glycogen reserves are converted into glucose, and the eye pupils dilate. Adrenaline secretion is produced by motor impulses directly from the brain, and nerves from the sympathetic nervous system stimulate the secretory cells of the medulla to release it. Since little of our anxiety is linked to life or death survival situations, continual stress can tax the adrenals and sympathetic nervous system.

This link between the brain and adrenaline stimulation illustrates well the effect our emotions can have on the hormonal balance in our bodies.

Islets of Langerhans in the Pancreas

These are clusters of endocrine tissue in the pancreas, rather than a separate gland. The regulation of blood sugar levels in the blood is regulated by insulin, the main hormone produced by these glands. Insulin reduces the level of glucose in the blood by accelerating its conversion to glycogen in the liver. It also regulates the uptake of sugar by the tissues of the body. A failure of sugar absorption due to insufficient insulin results in high blood sugar levels, sugar in the urine, and the inability of the body to use sugar for energy, leading to weight loss. This is diabetes mellitis.

Excessive insulin leads to hypoglycemia, which is glucose insufficiency. Glucagon helps to break down the glycogen stored in the liver, which releases more sugar into the blood. It also assists lipid and protein metabolism. Glucagon secretion can be stimulated by stress and exercise.

Ovaries and Testes

The ovaries produce the female hormones estrogen and progesterone in response to the pituitary hormones FSH and LH. These control the menstrual cycle, and in the case of fertilization of the egg, maintain a suitable environment for its implantation. Estrogen dominates the first half of the cycle, progesterone the second half, and both are involved throughout pregnancy. FSH and LH also control the ripening and release of ova.

The testes have two functions in the male: development and excretion of spermatazoa, and production and secretion of the male sex hormone testosterone. Secretory cells in the testes produce testosterone in response to the stimulation of luteinizing hormone produced by the pituitary gland. Testosterone helps the production of sperm, and in the development of male secondary sex characteristics at puberty: body hair, changes in voice, skeletal growth, growth of penis, and libido.

Now that we have looked at the structure and function of the endocrine system in fairly conventional terms, there are a few other theories you should know about.

Olfaction and the Endocrine System

This is an area that can be potentially important for aromatherapists. In the chapter on olfaction we discussed briefly the link between pheromones and sexual behavior. Hormones are secreted within the organism, but pheromones are secreted into the environment. In animals, we know that the scent secreted is absolutely compelling, and is directly related to hormonal cycles and sexual activity. It is not so simple with humans, but we know that just before ovulation women are much more sensitive to certain odors such as musk, and their sense of smell on the whole is more acute at this time. We also know that pregnant women are acutely sensitive to certain odors.

An interesting sidelight to this, and to the issue of oils not suitable for pregnancy, is my own experience when I was pregnant, working every day bottling orders for oils. I found I couldn't stand smelling the oils that weren't good for me at that time. These were generally the stronger oils such as thyme, marjoram, rosemary, basil, peppermint, etc. They even smelled different. The only way I could cope was by wearing a vapor mask so I couldn't smell them at all.

I had planned to use certain oils during my labor, but couldn't handle any strong oils then, either. After the birth I found lavender very comforting, but it took a while to regain any real appreciation for my beloved essences.

I've also noted that many women are attracted to specific odors at different phases of their menstrual cycle. Clary sage seems very comforting during actual menstruation, and the aphrodisiac oils are often appealing during ovulation.

So our hormonal balance can affect our ability to smell, as well as our sensitivity to certain types of odors. It is true that many people with a diminished sense of smell also have a diminished libido.

The length of the menstrual cycle has been linked to olfactory contact between men and women; we know that body scent is a strong attracting factor between individuals, and that a woman's body scent changes, depending on the point she is in her menstrual cycle. Men often can detect this.

The apocrine and the eccrine, or sweat glands, are the main agents for carrying body scent. In 1886, French psychologist Auguste Galopin wrote, "...the purest marriage that can be contracted between a man and a woman is that engendered by olfaction."

Another point to note is that in early man an acute sense of smell was necessary for detecting enemies and danger. Detecting danger must have alerted the "fight or flight" response, which triggers adrenaline release and all the other responses that originate in the adrenal medulla.

Olfaction influences our hormonal state in other ways. There is a link between the limbic system and the hypothalamus, which we know is directly linked to the endocrine system through the pituitary. We know that the pituitary affects the sexual glands in the secretion of their hormones, and also affects the adrenal glands, which play a big part in coping with stress.

Tisserand directly links inhalation of aromatic molecules with the release of certain neurochemicals, and emotional responses. He says that oils which are mood regulators, and which help with anxiety, depression, mood swings, and menstrual/menopausal imbalances, affect the hypothalamus, and lists oils such as bergamot, frankincense, geranium, and rosewood as being especially effective. Aphrodisiac oils are thought to particularly affect the pituitary, and to stimulate release of the neurochemical endorphins, which are painkillers but also induce feelings of euphoria and heightened sexuality. He lists clary sage, jasmine, patchouli, and ylang-ylang as important.

Experience indeed shows that these are strong aphrodisiacs. One of my clients wanted to conceive a baby. She discovered she that became sexually aroused immediately upon smelling rose oil. So she and her husband made rose oil their nightly anointment; he also took a large dose of ginseng. Following these steps she became pregnant within two months. They seriously considered naming their new daughter "Rose"!

Specific oils are known to influence specific glands. This explains to a large extent their effectiveness as aphrodisiacs, although we also know that certain oils help to bring circulation, warmth, and relaxation to the sexual areas. Some relax the nervous system to help get rid of anxiety, some provide emotional effects, and so forth. A beautiful scent can be romantic, and some oils deal with the adrenaline levels which can help or hinder the ability to reach orgasm. Scent can also bring back memories of a romantic time, or create a bond for future memories. As we know, sexuality is much more than a question of genitals; because there are so many factors involved, we cannot cover them all here.

The Essential Oils and the Endocrine System

Essential oils can affect the hormonal balance in the body directly or indirectly. As a direct action, the oils work as phytohormones, in the same way that an animal or human hormone would work on the body. Sometimes the plant hormone will be found in the oil, such as estrogen in clary sage, sometimes in another part of the plant. Herbalists make use of many plants in this way. For example, willow tree catkins are a good source of plant estrogen.

Oils and herbal preparations may also act indirectly, by triggering a particular gland into action or by balancing its hormonal secretion in some way. Gumbel[1] makes the statement that "…the latest scientific test results show that the effect mechanisms of essential oils are—if not the same—at least similar to those of hormones. Also the chemical combination of both is in many cases extraordinarily similar to each other." He goes on to talk about estrogen-like and androgen-like substances in plants, such as the estrogenic action of hops and sage and the androgenic action of parsley.

Valnet[2] also calls attention to the hormonal effects of plants, citing an article called "Vegetable Hormones" written by Decaux in 1961, in which he called attention to the fact that certain vegetable substances contain sexual hormones. Valnet says this is important to know in all therapy, because using certain plants may cause hormonal imbalances. He also says, "…the essence is to the plant as hormones are to the endocrine glands." They seem to have balancing and stimulating effects on the endocrine glands. Valnet cites cypress as being a homologue of the ovarian hormone, and says that pine needle will stimulate the adrenal cortex. Following is a list of the glands and the oils specific to each.

Pituitary: Restorer: sage. *General:* clary sage, jasmine, patchouli, ylang-ylang, ginseng.

Oxytocin stimulants: General: myrrh, sage, lavender, jasmine (lavender and jasmine are used in labor, but they are not proven oxytocins).

Pineal: General: sage.

Thyroid: Balancers: garlic, onion. *Restorer:* parsley. *General:* ginseng.

Parathyroids: Restorer: juniper.

Thymus: General: tea-tree, eucalyptus.

Adrenals: Cortical hormone stimulants: pine, savory, thyme, rosemary. *Cortical hormone inhibitor:* ylang-ylang. *Medulla stimulants:* basil, geranium, lemon, pine, rosemary, savory, thyme. *Medulla inhibitor:* ylang-ylang. *Adrenal gland restorers:* juniper, parsley, ginseng.

Pancreas: Restorers: black pepper, fennel, juniper.

Insulin stimulants: General: carrot, eucalyptus, fennel, geranium, lemon, onion, sage.

Ovaries: Restorer: parsley. *General:* ginseng. *Estrogen stimulants:* aniseed, angelica, camomile, cypress, fennel, geranium, rosemary, clary sage, sage. *Estrogen inhibitor:* cumin. *Progesterone stimulants:* lady's mantle, sarsaparilla, yarrow (used as an herbal infusion).

Testes: Testosterone stimulants: lemon, parsley, savory, ginseng.

Gonadatropic hormones regulator: General: sage.

Mammary glands: Galactagogues: caraway, aniseed, fennel, dill, jasmine. *To stop milk:* cypress, geranium, peppermint, sage.

The Endocrine Glands and Chakras

Shafica Karagulla and Dora van Gelder Kunz[3] have discussed the relationship between certain disease processes and the chakras. Dora van Gelder Kunz developed "Therapeutic Touch" with Dolores Krieger, and has worked with many medical people, teaching them how to utilize the subtle energy fields of the human body for healing. The chakras have been used for thousands of years in Indian and Tibetan medicine. Van Gelder Kunz defines them as "…superphysical centers or organs through which the energies of the different

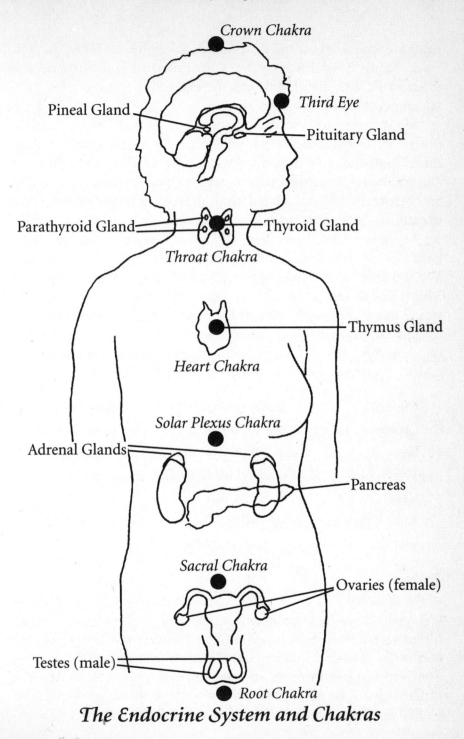

The Endocrine System and Chakras

fields are synchronized and distributed to the physical body." In their book, Karagulla and van Gelder Kunz link certain disturbances of the chakras with disturbances in the endocrine gland related to it, and cite case histories to back this up.

Many people who receive various kinds of body work or chiropractic treatment find they improve for a short time after the treatment, but slide right back. Progress is gradual, but slow. A chiropractor I've worked with balances the chakra in a particular area before the adjustment, and finds that once the body is balanced, the adjustments seem much more effective.

I believe essential oils definitely act on the subtle bodies, and I have worked with specific oils in relation to specific chakras. I usually add an oil that relates to the specific gland for that chakra, and have found this to be a useful approach. This may be something you would like to pursue, as these links are all tentative at this time.

On the following page is a table of the commonly accepted correlations between the chakras and the endocrine glands. I have added suggestions for corresponding essential oils.

Chakra	Endocrine Gland	Essential Oil
Crown	Pineal	Frankincense
Brow	Pituitary	Sandalwood
Throat	Parathyroid/thyroid	Lavender
Heart	Thymus	Rose
Solar Plexus	Adrenals/pancreas	Ginger
Sacral	Ovaries and testes	Jasmine
Root	Spine/glandular system	Vetivert

In working with students, I have found that opinions vary widely about which oils correspond with which chakras. I have suggested an oil for each chakra, but there are many possibilities. Try meditating on the different chakras and glands and see what you come up with. Remember, when working with the chakras you are working on a different level, so the oils that correspond with the physical gland will be different, although I think that working with both therapeutically would be stronger than working on just one level. You can, of course, just work with the oils and glands on a physical level.

The Endocrine Glands and Reflexology

I have included reflexology in the discussions of the different body systems because I think that using the zones of the feet, and even different oils for different body systems, can be a wonderful addition to any massage you are doing. The endocrine system can be influenced through the reflexes in the feet by using oils specific to the glands you are working with. One reflexologist I know routinely stimulates menstruation, and in some cases even labor, by working with these areas. Once again, I advise caution in using oils or any techniques mentioned in this book if you have not been fully trained in the method being considered.

Endnotes

1. Gumbel, G. *Principles of Holistic Skin Therapy with Herbal Essences.* Heidelberg, Germany: Haug, 1986.

2. Valnet, J. *The Practice of Aromatherapy.* Saffron Walden, England: C. W. Daniel, 1980.

3. Karagulla, S. and D. van Gelder Kunz. *The Chakras and the Human Energy Fields.* Wheaton, Illinois: Theosophical Publishing House, 1989.

11

Performing a Consultation

In this final chapter we will examine the process of conducting an aromatherapy consultation and determining an individual blend. We will then discuss the issues involved in setting yourself up as an aromatherapy consultant, professional ethics, and what it means to be a practicing aromatherapist.

Once you have internalized the information presented in the preceding chapters and have an intimate knowledge of the oils through living, working, and learning with them, you will know which oils will be appropriate in various situations without having to go through the process of listing, cross referencing, eliminating, and so forth that we described earlier. However, no matter how extensive your knowledge of aromatherapy is or may become, it is always important to spend some time in consultation with each client before you mix the oils. There are many issues that you must consider, and many things that you can observe if you take the time with each person. The consultation is designed to get a complete physical, mental, emotional, and spiritual picture of the person before you. This picture will help you to choose a range of oils that will be appropriate for this particular person at this particular time.

You will be amazed at how much your clients will progress if they are using the right oils in the right way. At times the rate of change will seem miraculously rapid, but in other cases you will need to persevere to see any real change. Be observant, encourage them to be observant, and please develop the habit of keeping records of the oils you use and the results you get. This should also be done by your client, as his or her perceptions will be different from yours.

Please note that if the oils are doing their job, change will occur, and each time you see the client you probably will need to go through the process again. Don't make up one blend that is used without change; you will need to adjust it from time to time. Furthermore, it is not advisable to use one oil continuously in excess for an extended period. The properties of the oils overlap enough that you can and should change them regularly.

Before the client arrives, make sure your room or office is attractive, clean, and cheerful. Use color and lighting to create the atmosphere you wish to convey, and flowers are always a nice addition. You might have a burner on with an appropriate oil, or you may choose to spray the room with an aromatherapy air spray. Prepare yourself for the consultation by centering, calming, cleansing, and protecting yourself. Everyone has their own method for doing this, through breathing, repeating a mantra, imagining cleansing images such as a waterfall or protecting images such as a white light surrounding oneself. You owe it to yourself and your client to do this. Soft music may be appropriate, and you may wish to take the phone off the hook.

I think that the way that you dress is important. When I first arrived in the United States, from England, I was shocked to see massage therapists working in T-shirts and jogging pants, as I was trained to always wear a professional-looking white uniform. Although America is more informal, and we cannot represent ourselves as medical persons, I do think it is important to look professional when we are working with clients, particularly if we want aromatherapy eventually to be recognized as a profession. People will have more confidence in what you have to offer if you look the part and conduct yourself accordingly.

I normally set aside about 30 minutes for a consultation. If you are not going to give a treatment such as a massage, this is usually enough to go through the consultation process and help the client choose oils that would be appropriate. Charge a consultation fee which is comparable with those charged by other health professionals in your area.

Remember that you can choose whom you see. Do not be pressured into working with someone if you feel instinctively wary of the person, or it is not convenient for you to see them at that particular time. Don't be afraid to say "No," and don't be bullied into doing a consultation by telephone, or making up oils for someone you have never seen. You will regret it, and could end up in trouble. You must see the person before you can choose appropriate oils. I get letters from people asking what oils would be good for their eczema, for example, and I always reply that I work only through personal consultation, as each case is individual, and each person will need a unique blend of oils.

You may think camomile would be great for eczema, and send a big bottle of it through the mail. What if that person is allergic to camomile and the rash gets worse? Also, you do not know who you are dealing with. If the person is not serious enough to make an appointment to see you, he or she is not serious enough about changing his or her situation or state of health. Use your time and energy wisely and professionally; if you respect yourself, others will respect you.

Many of you will wonder why I am saying all of this. It seems obvious, and if you are already a therapist you will know it already. I know all of it too, but I still get drawn into situations I don't want, forget to take time to prepare myself adequately for a consultation, take on others' burdens, fail to say "No" when I should, and so on, so there is no harm in reminding ourselves of these things.

The Consultation

Let's say that the client has arrived and we are ready to begin. First you will record your client's name, address, phone number, occupation, marital status, and date of birth on your form. Many practitioners have a questionnaire which clients fill out themselves, but I have always found that by going through the questionnaire with them I get far more information than if they merely tick boxes or write comments without elaborating or giving me any more insight into their character.

I like to have the date of birth rather than age, because some people object to giving their age, and asking for birth date does not seem so threatening. Also, because I have observed some truth in astrology, it lets me know what birth sign they are. This often correlates with the type of oils they like; for example, earth types often like the heavier earthy or woody oils, while fire types like the hotter oils. Even if you get only an idea of the element, it is useful and gives you another little insight into their character.

The client's marital status can give you clues to his or her emotional state; the occupation can tell you about his or her educational background, lifestyle, and self-image. Sometimes you can also get some idea of his or her personality type and psychological profile.

I would then ask about the client's medical history, specifically about any of the conditions that would contraindicate the use of certain oils, for example epilepsy or pregnancy. Asking what type of treatment he or she has received in the past also tells you about his or her attitude toward health, and openness to what you have to offer.

If the client is presently receiving treatment from another practitioner, it is important that you not interfere with that process. If you have any doubt, you should contact the practitioner and discuss what you are proposing. If still in doubt, keep away, and ask the client to come back after the treatment is finished.

Of course, it is important to ask what he or she hopes to work on with you, and why he or she is here today. Why a person chooses aromatherapy is often illuminating too. How did he or she find out about you? What does he or she know about the oils?

You can then go on to explain how the oils are believed to work, how many levels he or she can work on at once, and the different ways in which the oils can be used. This gives you an opening to explore the deeper dimensions of the problem, if this is appropriate. For example, if the problem is recurrent migraines, you could go into the nature of the headaches, their frequency, how long the condition has been occurring, and what medication your client may be taking for the pain.

You could then go on to look at physical causes such as diet or PMS, and then psychological and emotional factors like pressure from the boss at work or a husband who is having an affair.

All of the factors involved will determine which blend of oils you finally choose. You will also need to take into account the relative importance of each factor to the client. In the end, dealing with her fears and sense of betrayal because of her husband's affair, and recovering her own sexual self-confidence, may be more important for your client to work on with the oils than the actual migraines, although of course the oils also can help with the physical pain. This is where the individual blend is crucial in holistic aromatherapy. While we are helping with the headache, we are also helping to rebalance the whole person on many levels. If this is not done, the headaches will come back, no matter how many painkillers she takes. Of course, the beauty of the oils is that without consciously blending for all of these levels, a single oil will often do this anyway. For example, lavender would help the pain, both physically and emotionally.

Alternatively, if your client replies that the problem is depression and apathy, you may want to ask questions which will help to determine on what other levels this is operating. For example, Mr. Jones may be cold physically, he may be constipated, and may suffer indigestion. You could use oils to warm both body and spirit, selecting them by the three-column blending method described earlier.

Sometimes you will simply want to use the oils on a physical level, such as making a facial blend for a mature dry skin, and will use one oil as an antiwrinkle aid, one for broken capillaries, and one as a sebum balancer. However, factors such as diet and hormonal balance will still come into play.

You may also blend for purely spiritual purposes, for example, creating a blend that will deepen breathing, open the third eye, and calm the mind. One day someone may ask you to create a personal perfume; in this case your three columns might be concerned with picking top, middle, and base notes.

Thus, the reason why a person is consulting you will determine your next set of questions. I would have a set of questions covering the main body systems, and a set covering all types of stress. You don't have to ask everything, just use what is appropriate.

Once you have concluded your questionnaire, have your client sign a disclaimer assuming full responsibility for using the oils. This will protect you, particularly since it is illegal for us as unlicensed practitioners to prescribe, diagnose, or treat any medical condition. We cannot say, "This camomile oil will help your eczema," or "I want you to apply this rosemary to the area of your liver three times a day," or "It sounds like your have exhausted adrenal glands."

Once you have determined which oils you think would be applicable, the best thing to do is to present them to the client, and let him or her choose the ones he or she feels most drawn to. You don't have to explain in detail why you have chosen them, although you can refer to the commonly accepted use of each oil: "Camomile has been traditionally used as an anti-inflammatory oil," or to what an authority says: "Tisserand speaks of tea-tree as a booster of the immune system." You could also refer to research: "There has just been a study by Australian scientists which showed that tea-tree was effective against candida in 85 percent of cases." You can also refer to your own experience: "I found tea-tree very useful when I had candida." Do not say, "I want you to use this tea-tree three times a day as a treatment for your candida."

Having made the blend, you can give it to your client with a list of accepted means of using the oils and instructions for how much oil to use for each, so that he or she has general instructions for use. Do not write on the bottle, "Add eight drops of rosemary oil to your bath twice a day." Your sheet might say, "The recommended amount of essential oil to use in a bath is six to eight drops."

If you approach your consultation and the administering of the oils in this way, you will not be accused of practicing medicine without a license, and if you have your clients sign the disclaimer, thus taking responsibility for their own health, you are merely acting as an advisor or consultant.

It is best to call yourself an aromatherapist or aromatherapy consultant. As yet, there is no licensing or regulation of aromatherapy or the use of oils in the United States. We can use them because they appear on the list of GRAS (generally recognized as safe) food additives published by the U.S. Food and Drug Administration (FDA). As of this writing, the FDA has no plans to interfere with the use of oils for psychological purposes, and will approach other aromatherapeutic uses on a case-by-case basis. If drug-like claims are made openly, this could attract unwanted attention, so we must be very careful about how we represent ourselves as practitioners. The National Association for Holistic Aromatherapy is studying the establishment of training and professional standards for all of us. It is much better that we regulate ourselves rather than have strict regulations imposed on us.

If you are already a massage therapist, cosmetologist, acupuncturist, chiropractor, physician, registered nurse, or any other licensed professional, you can use the oils within your established practice. Licensing requirements differ widely from state to state, so if you wish to do hands-on work, or massage, and do not have a license, it is important that you determine your local requirements. Please check with your local authorities and comply with the regulations for the area in which you live.

Ethics

This is a complicated issue—everyone has their own values. However, I believe that it is very important for us to have our own code of ethics as aromatherapy practitioners. One of the most important considerations is to work within your own limits. Do not pretend to know more than you do, and use the oils in a responsible, humble way. Do not underestimate their power, and let them teach you about themselves by using them with respect, restraint and subtlety.

Too often I have seen the oils overused, over-blended, and causing damage, through the neglect of the people using them. Use them gently, with pride in your craft, and they will work wonders for you.

If we are to be holistic practitioners, we should respect the laws of nature, observe her patterns, and attempt to live in harmony with the earth. I hope you will strive to avoid excess commercialism and exploitation of aromatherapy and the essential oils. These remedies are not merely another product to be sold; they contain the life force itself. Be as simple and honest as possible in all of your dealings, and when recommending the oils to others, always err on the side of caution and restraint.

Practice what you preach, use the oils in your personal life, and try to speak from personal experience. Question everything until you have internalized the knowledge, and know what is true from your own experience and inner work. Strive for the very highest standards in your training and practice. Continue asking questions and growing in your knowledge. The more I use the oils, the more they teach me; if you let them, they will show you far more than any book, course, or teacher ever could.

Appendix:
The 24 Essential Oils

The life force of the plant, called by alchemists the soul or "quintessence," essential oils are found in roots, bark, stalks, leaves, resins, and flowers of certain plants and trees. The oils are secreted by special glands, ducts, or cells in one or more parts of the plant, and act as plant hormones. A plant generally contains a small quantity of essential oil, as little as a tenth to ten percent. The qualities of the oil may vary with different times of day and different seasons. Climate and growing location influence the ultimate chemical properties.

Within a plant, essences play a part in its development, help pollinization by attracting certain insects and birds, and protect against infection, bacteria, and fungi. They protect the plant from heat by evaporating from the leaf surfaces, and may also act as a selective weed killer.

Physical Characteristics

- Highly volatile, some more so than others. Differing evaporation rates and molecular sizes create a scale of "notes": top, middle, and base. Bottles containing essential oils should be capped when not in use.

- Highly concentrated, they must be diluted to prevent overdose. One drop is equivalent to 25 cups of herbal infusion; one drop of rose oil equals 30 roses.

- Sensitive to light and heat. Keep in dark glass bottles in even, moderate temperature.

- Will destroy some plastics and strip paint.

- Will dissolve in lipids or alcohol, not water.

- Not greasy.

- Shelf life of up to six years if stored correctly. (Absolutes and resins have a shorter shelf life.)

Therapeutic Properties

- Most essential oils are antiseptic, attacking bacteria and viruses, decomposing and neutralizing them.

- Some essential oils contain plant hormones, and antiseptics.

- They work synergistically. The more they are interfered with, the less their therapeutic effectiveness.

- They work in harmony with the vital forces of the body, to balance and correct underlying disharmonies rather than suppress the symptoms.

- Most oils are cytophylactic; they stimulate the growth of new cells and promote tissue formation.

Chemical Constituents

The properties of each essential oil depend on its chemical structure, although this comprises many different elements, an oil and its therapeutic effects can be categorized by its main chemical constituent:

- *Alcohols:* bactericidal, energizing, vitalizing, diuretic, antiviral.

- *Aldehydes:* anti-inflammative, calming, sedative, antiviral.

- *Esters:* spasmodic, fungicidal, anti-inflammative, effects central nervous system.

- *Cetones or Ketones:* wound healing, mucolytic, dermatophilic, lipophilic.

- *Phenols:* bactericidal, antifungal, immune-stimulant, invigorating, warming, skin irritant.

- *Sesquiterpenes:* anti-inflammative, antiviral, antiphlogistic.

- *Terpenes:* stimulant, potential irritant, antiviral.

Methods of Use and Recommended Dilutions

- *Baths:* six to eight drops in the bath, less with irritating oils such as lemon, peppermint, thyme.

- *Burners:* four to six drops in top of burner or potpourri simmerer.

- *Compresses:* six drops in bowl of hot or cold water, pick up with cloth, wring out, and apply to area.

- *Inhalations:* four drops in bowl of hot water.

- *Massage:* three percent solution—three drops in one teaspoon of carrier oil or 18 drops in one ounce carrier oil.

- *Carrier Oils:* apricot kernel, hazelnut, avocado, wheatgerm, canola, jojoba, sesame, evening primrose, grapeseed.

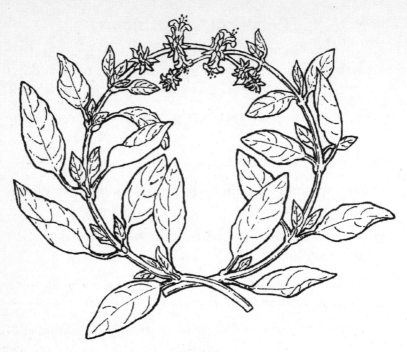

Basil

Latin name: Ocimum basilicum.

Botanical family: Lamiaceae.

Origins: Asia, North America, Reunion, France, Cyprus, Seychelles.

Part of plant used: Flowering tops and leaves.

Method of production: Distillation.

Evaporation rate: Top.

Chemical constituents: Phenol methylchavicol, linalol, camphor, cineol, eugenol, pinene.

Growing habits

Basil grows wild all over the Mediterranean, and has been grown in England since the sixteenth century. It is a bushy annual, two to three feet tall, with a squarish stem, numerous branches, shiny, green-toothed, inch-long leaves, and blooms from June to September.

Plant lore

The word *basilicum* comes from the Greek, and means "royal." It was considered the king of herbs. Its seeds were used in Galenic and Persian medicine, and it was thought that for the plant to flourish, the planting had to be accompanied by cursing and foul language! In ancient Egypt, basil leaves were scattered over graves. Basil is a sacred plant, *ocimum sanctum,* to the Hindus, and was grown in pots near temples and outside almost every house. It is dedicated to the gods Vishnu and Krishna and is used extensively in Ayurvedic medicine. The roots were made into beads and worn around necks and arms, the seeds made into rosaries. The leaves were placed on the breast of the dead, to help open the gates of heaven. Its rule by Mars and Scorpio well matches these tales.

Therapeutic qualities

Basil is thought of as a warming oil, although it has a cool quality like peppermint. Its best known actions are on the brain and digestive system. It has antiseptic, antidepressant, antispasmodic, carminative, cephalic, digestive, emmenagogic, expectorant, febrifuge, nervine, adrenal cortex stimulating, stomachic, sudorific, and tonic properties.

Practical applications

- *Blending.* Basil blends well with lavender, citrus, and geranium.

- *Brain and nervous system.* This is one of the classic applications of basil. It is a good remedy for headaches, migraines (also due to its soothing action on the digestive system), head colds, and in restoring the brain, nervous system, and adrenals in cases of extreme stress and exhaustion. It helps lift depression and clears a muddled brain. It may also help in coping with grief and anxiety.

- *Digestive system.* Basil's carminative action helps with nausea, vomiting, and spasmodic stomach pains.

- *Respiratory system.* Basil is a good antispasmodic remedy for coughing, wheezing, phlegm, coldness in the lungs. It is also effective in treating bronchitis, sinus congestion, and loss of the sense of smell.

- *Reproductive system.* As an emmenagogue, basil helps promote delayed or scanty menstruation, eases cramps, and combats infertility linked with emotional coldness or mental concerns.

- *Skin care.* Good for congested, toxic skin. It helps promote the circulation and warmth necessary to carry away waste products. It is a good tonic, but must be used with care and in weak dilution, because it can irritate sensitive skin. It also makes a good insect repellent.

- *Psychological effects.* Promotes clarity of thought and feeling. Uplifting and warm, soothes the troubled mind and heart.

Methods of use

- *Brain and nervous system.* Baths, burners, compresses for headaches, inhalations, massages, personal perfume.

- *Digestive system.* As a massage oil for the stomach and kidney area, compresses.

- *Respiratory system.* Burners, chest rubs, inhalations.

- *Skin care.* Very dilute massage oil, facial spray, compresses.

Further notes

I always think of basil as one of the cephalic trio. It has a pleasant, licorice odor, and somehow has a softer edge than peppermint or rosemary. It is penetrating without being quite so piercing.

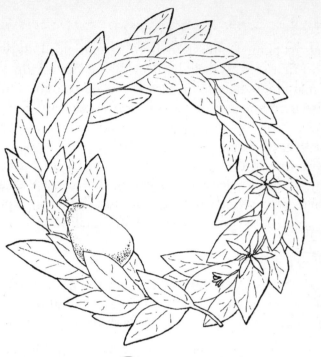

Bergamot

Latin name: Citrus bergamia.

Botanical family: Rutaceae.

Origins: Southern Italy, Ivory Coast, Guinea.

Part of plant used: Rind from small orange-like fruit.

Method of production: Expression; yield 0.5 percent.

Evaporation rate: Top.

Chemical constituents: Linalol, limonene, linalyle acetate, bergapten, bergamotin, camphene.

Growing habits

The oil used in aromatherapy should not be confused with the bergamot plant, which is an herb indigenous to North America. The tree grows to a height of 15 feet, and the fruits are picked from December to February.

Plant lore

The oil gets its name from the town of Bergamo in Italy, where the essence was first sold. Widely used in the perfume industry, bergamot is a main ingredient in the classic eau-de-cologne. Oil of bergamot is also used to flavor the favorite Earl Grey tea.

Therapeutic qualities

Bergamot is one of the most pleasant, uplifting oils used in aromatherapy. It has analgesic, antidepressant, antiseptic, antispasmodic, carminative, cicatrisant, deodorant, digestive, expectorant, febrifuge, sedative, vermifuge, and vulnary qualities.

Practical applications

- *Blending.* Bergamot blends well with the florals: rose, jasmine, neroli, lavender, and geranium. A blend of lavender, bergamot, and geranium is a lovely skin toner or perfume.

- *Nervous system.* Bergamot is a wonderfully uplifting antidepressant, and carries the cheer of all the citrus oils with a floral, warm, softer quality. It can be used for anxiety, nervous tension, in convalescence, and to help regulate eating disorders such as anorexia. It seems to affect the heart center and has marked sedative qualities. It also helps with insomnia. A lavender/bergamot blend is nice for this.

- *Digestive system.* Other classic uses for bergamot are controlling nausea, stimulating and regulating the digestion and liver, and helping to get rid of colic and flatulence.

- *Excretory system.* One of the best remedies for cystitis, leucorrhoea, urethritis, and vaginal pruritis, also a good excretory antiseptic.

- *Skin care.* Bergamot is an excellent antiseptic for cases of acne, oily skin, and infected skin conditions. Its aroma is beautifully suited for skin care as long as it is used in a very dilute form (one percent or less). However, the oil increases the photosensitivity of the skin, and it should not be used on skin areas which will be exposed to sunlight. It is an effective deodorant and insect repellent, and can be useful, in weak dilution, for seborrhoea, eczema, psoriasis, and wounds that fail to heal.

- *Immune system.* Effective against *herpes simplex,* and is a strong antiviral agent. It can be used to allay discomfort in cases of shingles and chicken pox. It is also useful in bringing down a fever. Tisserand says it is effective against gonococcus, staphylococcus, coli, meningococcus, diphtheria bacillus, and tuberculosis bacilli.

- *Reproductive system.* Some writers suggest it for uterine tumors and fibroids.

Methods of use

- *Nervous system.* Massage, baths, burners, personal perfume, inhaling oil from a handkerchief throughout the day.

- *Digestive system.* Massage oil rubbed over the abdomen.

- *Excretory system.* Sitz baths, baths, local wash or douche (very dilute, one percent or less). Massage oil over the lower abdomen and kidneys.

- *Skin care.* Add in low dilution to skin cream, oil or lotion. Do not use before exposure to sunlight. Toner: mix a few drops with two or three drops of lavender and a small amount of vodka (about a half teaspoon), add to a half pint distilled water or rose water. Can be used in compresses too.

- *Immune system.* Baths, burners, massage.

- *Reproductive system.* Sitz baths, local massage, compresses.

Further notes

Bergamot is one of the most beautiful of the citrus oils, and has a floral note reminiscent of neroli. It was the first essential oil I ever bought, and I used it as a perfume. We have to thank the perfume industry for bergamot's existence as an essential oil.

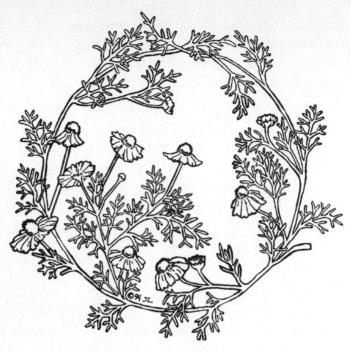

Camomile

Latin names: *Anthemis nobilis* (Roman camomile), *Matricaria chamomilla* (German camomile).

Botanical family: *Asteraceae.*

Origins: France, England, Morocco, Spain, Egypt, Belgium, Germany, Italy, Hungary.

Part of plant used: Flowers.

Method of production: Distillation; Roman yield is 0.5 to 1 percent, German yield is 0.22 to 0.23 percent.

Evaporation rate: Middle.

Chemical constituents: *Roman camomile:* angelate and butyate esters, a bitter principle, a special camphor, anthemene, sesquiterpenes (azulene, artemol), resin, gum phytosterol, calcium and sulphur. *German camomile:* ethers of caprylic and monylic acid, a hydrocarbon, and azulene. The main differences are that Roman camomile is strong on esters (60 to 80 percent); German camomile is strong in azulene (30 percent) and also contains oxides.

Growing habits

Camomile is fond of fields, lanes, gravel, dusty, stony land. It flowers from the beginning of July until the end of August, has daisy like-flowers and feathery leaves. German camomile (*Matricaria chamomilla*) is an annual, and grows between one and two feet tall. Roman camomile (*Anthemis nobilis*) is a perennial, and grows to about a foot high. Camomile has always been known as a good companion plant, and has been called "the plant's physician."

Plant lore

The name camomile, in Greek *chamoemelon*, means "earth apple," and this describes well camomile's earthy, yet sweet, and slightly tart aroma. The old Saxon word for camomile is *maythen;* it is one of the oldest known English herbs. In the language of flowers, camomile means "patience in adversity," and this is a good description for camomile's soothing qualities. It is said to be ruled by the sun, and is dedicated to St. Anne, mother of the Virgin Mary. Buckingham Palace has a camomile lawn in one of its gardens, and *Anthemis nobilis* means noble flower.

Therapeutic properties

Analgesic, antiallergic, anticonvulsive, antidepressive, antiphlogistic, antiseptic, antispasmodic, carminative, cholagogue, cicatrisant, digestive, diuretic, emmenagogic, febrifuge, hepatic, nervine, sedative, splenetic, stomachic, sudorfic, tonic, vasoconstrictor, vermifuge.

Practical applications

- *Blending.* Camomile tends to dominate a blend, so it is sometimes nice to add a drop of lavender, which softens its distinctive smell. *Matricaria* camomile is more bitter, and *Anthemis* more sweet. It blends well with geranium and rose. People seem either to love or hate camomile.

- *Nervous system.* Antidepressant, hysteria, sedative, eases insomnia, restlessness, nervous irritability, over-sensitivity, temper tantrums, anger (like rose, acts on the liver).

- *Digestive system.* Camomile's antispasmodic, digestive, and carminative qualities explain why it has been a favorite soothing digestive remedy for centuries. Camomile tea is famous for this. Used for dyspepsia, difficult digestion, flatulence, and gastric ulcers.

- *Excretory system.* Urinary and intestinal antiseptic, diuretic, good for cystitis, kidney stones, stimulates and restores the liver and spleen, helps leucocyte production.

- *Reproductive system.* Good for PMS, menstrual discomfort, irregular periods. *Matricaria chamomilla* is especially beneficial to women, and is called "The Mother Herb" because of this. Eases engorged breasts, mastitis, and menstrual problems linked to nervous disorders.

- *Muscles and joints.* A good analgesic for dull, continuous pain, particularly inflammation of the joints.

- *Inflammations.* Camomile is specifically anti-inflammatory because of its azulene content. It can be used to treat skin inflammation, children's teething, earaches, facial neuralgia, anything that is red or angry. Also used for conjunctivitis, sties (use camomile tea).

- *Children.* Camomile is one of the few oils safe to use on young children due to its low toxicity (use a one percent dilution) and it is good for most childhood diseases. It can also be used to gently lower intermittent fevers.

- *Skin care.* Good for sensitive skin, allergic rashes, dermatitis, chapped skin, broken capillaries, anti-inflammatory and promotes healing. Calming and gentle for even the most delicate of skin and for eczema.

Methods of use

- *Digestive system.* Camomile tea, abdomen compress, local massage.

- *Excretory system.* Baths, sitz baths, tea, squatting inhalations, local massage.

- *Reproductive system.* Baths, sitz baths, squatting inhalations, massage, douches (dilute, one percent), compresses.

- *Inflammations.* Lotions, compresses, baths; try to avoid direct massage.

- *Children.* Use in a very dilute form, about one percent. Avoid direct contact with eyes; if using for eye inflammation, use dilute camomile tea. Can be used in baths, massage, compresses, burners, inhalations. **Be careful!**

- *Skin care.* Lotions, oils, compresses, steaming (not for broken capillaries).

Further notes

Valnet writes as follows:

Azulene is a fatty substance discovered in the essence of *Matricaria* (camazulene). It possesses healing and antiphlogistic properties which have been studied chiefly by the Germans, and in France by Caujolle. Numerous experiments have shown its remarkable effectiveness in treating various inflammations of the skin, eczema, leg ulcers, vulvar pruritis, urticaria, and also chronic gastritis, colitis, cystitis, and certain kinds of asthma.

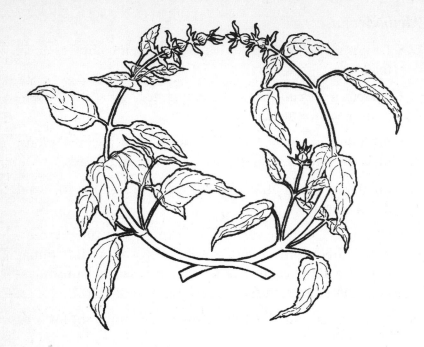

Clary Sage

Latin name: Salvia sclarea.

Botanical family: Lamiaceae.

Origins: Russia, Morocco, Southern France, United States, Syria.

Part of plant used: Flowering tops and foliage.

Method of production: Distillation.

Evaporation rate: Middle.

Chemical constituents: Borneol, salviol, cineol, sclareol, salvene, sclareol, and salvone.

Growing habits

Clary needs dry soil, and is a biennial plant which grows up to five feet tall. It has a large square stem, oval, finely toothed leaves and unusual, orchid-like, white, pale blue, or lilac flowers, with pink or lilac bracts. Clary flowers from May to September.

Plant lore

The name *sclarea* means "clear," and clary sage was often called "clear eye" in days gone by. Moistened seeds produce a mucilage which was used to wash the eyes and clear them of foreign matter. It was also used in making muscatel-like wine, because of its smoky, musty fragrance. However, the use of the essential oil with alcohol is ill-advised, as it seems to enhance the effect of alcohol and causes sickness, hangovers, and even nightmares. Robert Tisserand thinks that clary is euphoric, slowing the brain and causing cannabis-like effects. Because of clary's euphoric qualities, it is not a good idea to drive an automobile after its use.

Therapeutic qualities

Clary is anticonvulsive, antidepressive, antigalactagogic, antiseptic, antirheumatic, antispasmodic, antisudorific, aphrodisiac, astringent, carminative, deodorant, digestive, diuretic, emmenagogic, lymphatic, nervine, sedative, stomachic, tonic, and uterine.

Practical applications

- *Blending.* Lavender and clary is a deeply satisfying blend. Bergamot, orange, or mandarin are good companions from the citrus family. Jasmine and clary is a very sensual blend. Sandalwood or frankincense are also possible partners for clary. I'd bet clary and patchouli would be one weird blend, a real "love it or leave it."

- *Nervous system.* From the euphoric qualities of clary, you will have surmised that it has a strongly sedative effect on the nervous system. In fact, you could call clary one of the aromatherapy tranquilizes as are valerian and vetivert. I have noticed in classes that when students smell this oil, everyone immediately gets light-headed, drowsy, and starts speaking slowly, and not always coherently. It is usually at that point that we have to take a break for some fresh air! It is a wonderful oil for stress, helps with post-natal depression, is a nerve tonic to restore an exhausted nervous system, and seems to give one the space to switch off and heal oneself. Its euphoric quality helps uplift spirits even though the oil is so sedative. It is good in a migraine blend, and wonderful with lavender at night when an over-active mind keeps sleep at bay. Used without alcohol, it may even enhance your dream life in a positive way.

- *Muscular system.* Clary is a good muscle relaxant, and has strong antispasmodic qualities. It has a warming quality, and can help to deal both with the muscular tension itself and the stress and tension causing muscular spasm. I include clary in a blend when I want to create a "sledge-hammer" effect to knock the client out for an hour. It is one of the best remedies I know for menstrual cramps, and has an odor which fits well with female sexuality and gyneco-logical imbalances.

- *Reproductive system.* Clary, like rose otto, is a hormone bal-ancer, and so can be used to bring on late periods, or enhance scanty or difficult ones. It has a lot of plant estro-gen, so is useful in menopause when this hormone is on the decline, or any other period of feminine imbalance. It is useful to ease pain during labor and to help the mother relax. An aphrodisiac, clary is always a good addition to a blend for someone who is nervous, apprehensive, or overly analytical about sexual activity.

Methods of use

- *Nervous system.* Massage, baths, inhalations, burners or dif-fusers, personal perfume.

- *Muscular system.* Massage (full body or locally), compress, baths.

- *Reproductive system.* Massage over abdomen, lower back and tops of thighs; baths, compresses, inhalations during labor, sitz baths.

Further notes

I have found that clary is one of the oils that people either love or hate (like patchouli). It definitely has a very profound effect on people, and is one that many people crave at certain periods of their life. Many women find it deeply effective during or before their monthly cycle, and its scent has a strongly sexual side for an oil in the *lamiaceae* family. Sedative oils in reverse order of their strength would be lavender, marjoram, clary sage. Nobody could resist a blend of all three!

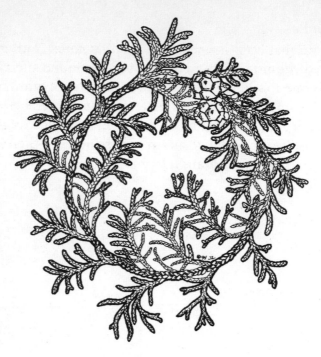

Cypress

Latin name: *Cupressus sempervirens.*

Botanical family: *Cupressaceae.*

Origins: Southern Europe, France, Germany, and Italy.

Part of plant used: Leaves and fruits ("cypress nuts").

Method of production: Distillation.

Evaporation rate: Middle to base.

Chemical constituents: Cymene (ketone), camphor of cypress, d-pinene, d-campene, d-sysvesterene, sabinol (terpenic alcohol), valeric acid.

Growing habits

Cypress is a perennial, tall, conical-shaped tree which has been used since antiquity. It can grow to a height of 66 feet, has short branches and small, scaly leaves. The male flowers are tiny; the female flowers are bright green, and grow into egg-shaped cones.

Plant lore

Cypress traditionally has been the tree of graveyards. Plato, alluding to its evergreen nature, said that it symbolized the immortality of the soul. The Persians believed it was originally the Tree of Paradise. The Greeks and Romans dedicated cypress to the gods of death and the underworld (Pluto and Hades), and the Egyptians used it for their sarcophagi because it was considered practically indestructible. *Sempervirens* means ever-living.

Therapeutic qualities

Antirheumatic, antispasmodic, antisudorific, astringent, deodorant, diuretic, hepatic, restorative of nervous system, styptic, vasoconstrictor.

Practical applications

Cypress is particularly good for any condition involving excess body fluids: edema, incontinence, excessive perspiration, bleeding gums, heavy menstrual flow, etc.

- *Blending.* Cypress blends well with juniper, lavender, pine, and sandalwood.

- *Reproductive system.* Menopausal problems, heavy periods, bleeding between periods, fibroids, hormonal imbalances. Stimulates endocrine secretion.

- *Circulatory system.* Astringent, stops hemorrhages, eases hemorrhoids and varicose veins. General system tonic.

- *Respiratory system.* Antispasmodic for bronchi, helps stop spasmodic coughing.

Methods of use

- *Reproductive system.* Baths, compresses, douches, massage.

- *Circulatory system.* Baths, massage.

- *Respiratory system.* Burners, chest rubs, inhalations, compresses.

Further notes

Juniper and cypress are related and share some of their properties. Juniper helps to release excess fluid, and cypress helps to stop it. Both work on body fluid levels; juniper is more diuretic, while cypress is more astringent.

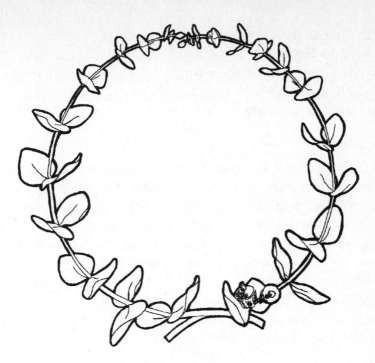

Eucalyptus

Latin name: Eucalyptus globulus (other chemotypes such as *Eucalyptus citriodora, Eucalyptus dives,* and *Eucalyptus radiata* are also used).

Botanical family: Myrtaceae.

Origins: Australia, Tasmania, Algeria, France, the Americas.

Part of plant used: Leaves.

Method of production: Distillation.

Evaporation rate: Top.

Chemical constituents: Eucalyptol, phellandrene, aromadendrene, eudesmol, pinene, camphene, valeric aldehydes.

Growing habits

Eucalyptus is one of the fastest growing trees in the world, reaching heights up to 480 feet. Because its huge root system absorbs vast amounts of water, it has been planted in marshy, malaria-infested areas to dry out the soil and purify the air. Eucalyptus flowers from November to December. It has highly aromatic leaves with a blue-green color, heart-shaped when young, long and lance-shaped when mature. There are more than 300 varieties of eucalyptus, and tea-tree comes from the same family. About 50 species yield a valuable oil.

Plant lore

The explorer and botanist Baron Ferdinand von Muller suggested in the 19th century that the fragrance of the tree might prove to be antiseptic. The French government sent seeds to Algeria during the 1850s, and many disease-ridden marshy areas were converted to healthy dry ones. The name eucalyptus means "well covered," which refers to the little cap which covers the flower bud before flowering, and *globulus* means "a little ball," which refers to the button-like form of the fruit. Eucalyptus has also been called the fever tree of Australia, the blue gum, and the woolly butt. The aborigines considered it a cure-all, and used the leaves to heal quite serious wounds.

Therapeutic qualities

Eucalyptus is analgesic, antiseptic, antispasmodic, cicatrisant, deodorant, depurative, diuretic, expectorant, febrifuge, hypoglycemiant, rebefacient, stimulant, vermifuge, and vulnerary.

Practical applications

- *Blending.* Eucalyptus is dominant in a blend, so if you don't want this effect, be careful of how much you add. It blends well with other tree oils such as pine, and the resins such as benzoin. Lavender is always a good friend.

- *Respiratory system.* One of the best remedies for the respiratory tract, it is antiseptic, expectorant, and antispasmodic. It helps to dry up phlegm, and combat sinusitis. It has also been indicated for emphysema, pneumonia, bronchitis, tuberculosis, asthma, coughs, and pulmonary congestion. Eucalyptus is said to have an antiviral action; air sprays containing it are highly effective in killing airborne bacteria.

When two of its chemical constituents, aromadendrene and phellandrene, contact the air they produce ozone, which makes it difficult for bacteria to survive. Eucalyptus, pine, and thyme make a good antiseptic and antibacterial mixture to disperse in the air in sickrooms. This mixture, with lavender added, is a good inhalation for bronchial conditions and throat infections.

- *Fevers.* Eucalyptus is of great help in lowering fever, in dealing with intermittent fevers, or conditions in which chills and fever alternate. Dilute eucalyptus can be applied in sponge baths, and the air saturated by air sprays and diffusers. Valnet mentions it as of particular use in malaria, typhus, measles, and scarlet fever. Patricia Davis also suggests it is useful in chicken pox.

- *Skin care.* Highly antiseptic, it is useful in treating burns and wounds, herpes, and shingles blisters. It is also effective as an insect repellent, in helping create new tissue, in removing tar from the skin, and as a deodorizer.

- *Urinary system.* Eucalyptus functions as a urinary antiseptic, helpful in urogenital infections such as cervicitis, cystitis, pyelitis, and nephritis. It is useful in clearing up vaginal infections involving discharge. It has a slight diuretic effect, and helps increase the excretion of urea.

- *Joints.* Because of its antirheumatic and antineuralgic qualities, it is also useful to add to rheumatic blends. It also is a rubefacient, and may be useful in increasing circulation and warmth to a painful joint.

- *Psychological effects.* Clears the mind, a breath of fresh air, reminds one of cleanliness, open spaces, cools fevers.

Methods of use

- *Respiratory system.* Inhalations, baths, chest and back rubs, compresses to the chest, diffusers.

- *Fevers.* Cool sponge baths.

- *Skin care.* Compresses, spraying dilute (one to two percent) oil onto the skin, baths, creams, and salves.

- *Genito-urinary system.* Sitz baths, local massage, pessaries for vaginal infections, dilute douches.

- *Joints.* Compresses, massage oils, baths.

Further notes

One of the most widely used and well-known oils, this is one to have in your home medicine chest, as well as your clinical bag, at all times. Almost all respiratory conditions can be treated by eucalyptus, as well as the viruses and bacteria that can trigger these problems. It is good to include eucalyptus in a blend when you know that someone will be more receptive to the oils used if the blend smells medicinal. Eucalyptus is a familiar smell for most people, which is reassuring when you are using oils they may not have experienced before.

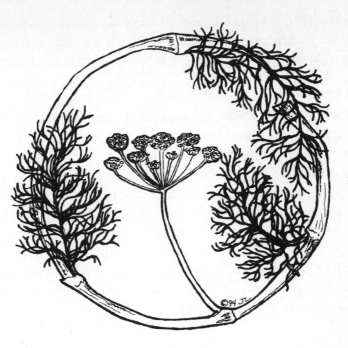

Fennel

Latin name: *Foeniculum vulgare.* *Foeniculum vulgare dulce* is the fennel grown as a vegetable.

Botanical family: *Apiaceae.*

Origins: Italy, California, India, Japan, Central Europe, England, the Mediterranean, and the coast of Wales.

Part of plant used: Crushed seeds.

Method of production: Distillation; yield 2.5 to 5 percent.

Evaporation rate: Middle.

Chemical constituents: Trans-anethole, fenchone, limonene, estragol, alpha pinene, myrcene, cineol, paracymene, pinene, anisaldehyde, camphene, cis-anethole, alpha phellandrene.

Growing habits

Fennel, a perennial, has bright green feathery leaves, and grows to approximately five to six feet high. It has yellow flowers which bloom from June to September. The seeds, which are actually fruits, are about a quarter inch long. Beekeepers often grow it as a honey plant.

Plant lore

Fennel is one of the oldest cultivated plants, and was highly esteemed by both the Greeks and Romans. The Greeks called it *marathon,* meaning to grow thin. Athletes ate it to give them energy without putting on weight, and Roman ladies ate it to keep from getting fat. Hippocrates and Dioscorides both mention it for the promotion of milk in nursing mothers. Pliny recommended it for physical eyesight and second sight, and it has long been considered a magical herb. Charlemagne decreed in 812 A.D. that it should be grown in all Imperial gardens. In medieval England, it was used to ward off witchcraft and evil spirits, and was chewed on fasting days to ward off hunger. It is dedicated to St. John the Baptist.

Therapeutic properties

Antiseptic, antispasmodic, antitoxic, carminative, diuretic, emmenagogic, laxative, sphlenetic, stomachic, tonic.

Practical applications

- *Blending.* Fennel generally dominates a blend, so if you want to go wholeheartedly with the sweet, aniseed smell, blends of seeds like cumin, coriander, aniseed, and fennel are generally successful. Other than that, you will smell fennel in any blend that contains it. Hot oils such as black pepper would be strong enough to counteract it, and could make an interesting combination.

- *Digestive system.* One of four traditional warming seeds (with aniseed, caraway, and coriander), it is a tonic to the digestion, liver, and spleen, is antispasmodic, dries mucous in the intestines, stops flatulence, helps appetite regulation, rids toxins from the system, helps nausea, indigestion, colic, and hiccups. Fennel tea is good for internal consumption.

- *Urinary system.* A diuretic, urinary tract antiseptic, fights urine retention, kidney stones, and uric acid in urine.
- *Antivenom, antipoison.* Helps remove toxins from the circulatory system, is an antidote for poisonous herbs and mushrooms and alcohol poisoning.
- *Endocrine system.* Helps correct irregular or scanty menstruation and estrogen insufficiency, helps the body to produce estrogen. Contraindicated for women with breast or reproductive system cancer, women who are taking contraceptive pills, and pregnant women. Encourages the production of breast milk and is helpful in relieving engorged breasts.
- *Gums.* Strengthens gums, hence its use in toothpaste.

Methods of use

- *Digestive system.* Using fennel and other seed oils in infusions is a good way to use fennel internally. Massage or using compresses over the abdomen and intestines is also effective.
- *Urinary system.* Infusions, baths, massage, and compresses over the kidneys.
- *Antivenom.* Use internally as infusion, or in an emergency, three or four drops in honey.
- *Detoxifying:* Baths, massage, lymphatic work, cellulite treatments.
- *Endocrine system.* Massage, baths, local compresses, massage, teas.
- *Gums.* Mouthwash (a few drops in warm water).

Further notes

Fennel is one of the most useful oils to use when working with the digestive or endocrine systems, and fennel tea is one of the most useful of the herbal infusions. Considered hot and dry, it seems to have an effect on the fluid mechanisms of the body.

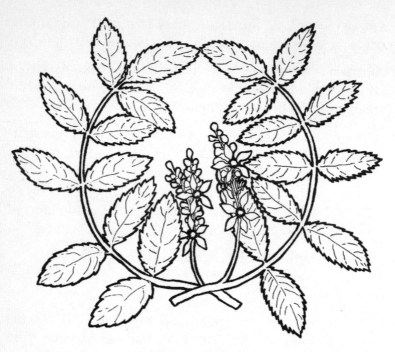

Frankincense (also known as olibanum)

Latin name: *Boswellia carteri.*

Botanical family: *Burseraceae.*

Origins: East Africa, Southern Arabia, Iran, and Lebanon.

Part of plant used: Resin.

Method of production: Distillation; yield four to seven percent.

Evaporation rate: Base.

Chemical constituents: L-pinene, dipentene, phellandrene, camphene, olibanol and various resins.

Growing habits

Frankincense is a small tree which grows in hot, dry climates. It has compact leaves and flowers which require little water. The whole plant is aromatic, and all parts have been burned for incense.

Plant lore

Frankincense is known as one of the sacred plants of antiquity. In the ancient world, frankincense, gold, and myrrh were the three most valuable substances known to man, and were offered by the three wise men in the Bible to baby Jesus in recognition of his divinity. It has always been associated with religious worship, and was originally used as incense. Considered to purify the surroundings of evil spirits, it is still used in Orthodox churches. *Frank* means "luxurious" in French, and *encens* means "incense." It is often simply called incense. The name *olibanum* is thought to derive from the Latin for "Oil from Lebanon."

Therapeutic qualities

Frankincense is antiseptic, astringent, carminative, cicatrisant, digestive, diuretic, sedative, tonic, uterine, and vulnary.

Practical applications

- *Blending.* Frankincense blends well with the other resins, like myrrh, woods like sandalwood, spices, and citrus oils.

- *Respiratory system.* Like eucalyptus, frankincense has a positive effect on the respiratory system. It is a good expectorant, and has a soothing and drying effect on mucous membranes. It is warm and dry, and thus is good for all excesses of phlegm, whether it is in the lungs, stomach, or bowels. Patricia Davis says that one of its main functions is in slowing and deepening the breathing, and this is why it is so useful in meditation and spiritual practice. Its antiseptic properties make it useful for pulmonary infections, and it is also useful in treating asthma.

- *Skin care.* Frankincense was used extensively for skin care in ancient Egypt and Greece. Some writers say it was used in embalming. It is known to help slow the effects of aging on the skin, and is an excellent rejuvenating treatment for older skin.

- *Circulatory system.* Its astringent qualities make this oil a good remedy for excessive bleeding of any kind.

- *Psychological effects.* Frankincense has always been used in this realm. It is a psychic cleanser and a good oil to burn when you want to clear the area around you from discordant vibrations. It helps one towards the light, and seems to open the higher chakras. It definitely elevates the mind, spirit, and emotions, and is said to be excellent for cutting ties and memories that bind one to the past. It helps rid one of obsessions, fear, and anxieties, and to put one's faith in something higher. I often use it when I feel disconnected from the spirit, or feel someone suffers from lack of faith.

Methods of use

- *Respiratory system.* Chest rubs, inhalations, compresses, baths, diffusers.

- *Skin care.* Lotions, facial massage oils, inhalations, masks.

- *Psychological effects.* Burners, diffusers, baths, massage.

Further notes

I cannot help but feel that this oil is something special. It speaks of centuries of devotion, spiritual aspiration and belief, and carries the magic of unknown realms. It is an aroma one remembers deep in the soul, and is a well of healing water in periods of doubt and when surrounded by materialism and superficiality.

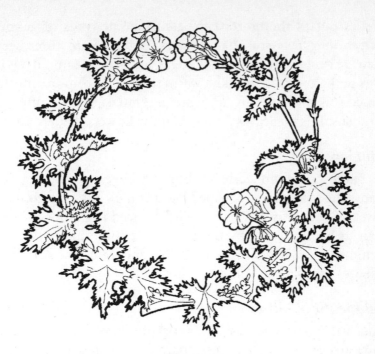

Geranium

Latin name: Pelargonium odorantissimum, and other varieties: *Pelargonium graveolens* (also *Pelargonium capitatum*) or rose geranium.

Botanical family: Geraniaceae.

Origin: Algeria, Reunion, Madagascar, and Guinea.

Part of plant used: Whole plant.

Method of production: Steam distillation.

Evaporation rate: Middle to top.

Chemical constituents: Geraniol, citronellol, linalol, terpineol, and alcohol.

Growing habits

Pelargoniums grow between three to four feet high in a herb garden, but are also grown as house plants. Only the scented *Pelargonium* is used for distilling essential oil, and there are about seven different varieties out of the more than 700 different types of geraniums. *Pelargoniums* have soft, hairy leaves, divided into three sections, which are deeply cut around the edges, and rose geranium has lavender or pink flowers. They like a warm sheltered position, moist, well-drained soil, and full sun. They are perennials, but are often grown as annuals. It is the leaves rather than the flowers that are aromatic.

Plant lore

The name geranium derives from the Greek *geranos* or "crane" because the seed pods are shaped like a crane's bill. Pelargoniums are native to South Africa. They were introduced to Europe in 1690 and began to be cultivated by the French perfume industry for "rose geranium oil." This is often used to adulterate rose oil. Culpeper attributes the plant to Venus.

Therapeutic qualities

Tonic, astringent, haemostatic, antiseptic, antidiabetic, anticancer, cicatrisant, antiseptic, analgesic, parasiticide, insect repellent, antidepressant, diuretic, adrenal cortex stimulant, hormone balancer.

Practical applications

- *Blending.* Two of the favorite partners of geranium are lavender and bergamot, and the three make a lovely blend. It also blends well with jasmine and rose, and the citrus oils bring out the sharp note in geranium.

- *Skin conditions.* Geranium is antiseptic, anti-inflammatory, good for eczema, wounds that are weeping and will not heal, burns and ulcers, is astringent without drying, demulcent, and soothing to mucous membranes. It balances sebum production in skin, so is good for all skin types. Also good as an insect repellent.

- *Circulatory system.* Geranium is haemostatic, making it useful in stopping hemorrhages (i.e., nosebleeds, injuries, or heavy menstrual periods). It is a tonic for the spleen.

- *Nervous system.* Antidepressant, not sedative as some people say; in fact, I have found geranium to be quite stimulating.

- *Endocrine system.* Has a stimulating effect on the adrenal cortex, which helps to balance hormones such as the sex hormones, so is indicated when the hormonal system is unbalanced. Valnet cites it as antidiabetic; it seems to work to balance the pancreas and blood sugar levels. Excessive breast milk and congestion of the breasts can be relieved with geranium. As an astringent, it also relieves excessive perspiration.

- *Reproductive system.* Helps produce estrogen and relieves fluid retention before the menstrual period. Relieves uterine hemorrhage, possibly works on uterine tumors.

- *Excretory system.* Helps with fluid retention, is a kidney tonic; useful in cellulitis treatments. As an excretory antiseptic, reduces diarrhea and mucous in stools and urine. Helps relieve bladder stones, jaundice, and is a liver tonic.

Methods of use

- *Skin.* Lotions, oils, compresses, baths, facials.
- *Circulatory system.* Baths, general and local massage.
- *Nervous system.* Baths, massage, inhalations.
- *Endocrine system.* Baths, general and local massage, compresses, inhalations.
- *Reproductive system.* Baths, douches, compresses, massage over endocrine glands, sitz baths.
- *Excretory system.* Massage over organs, baths, compresses.

Further notes

I always think of geranium as the great balancer. It seems to have a quality of equalizing hormonal and emotional extremes, and it seems to stand in the middle between flower and leaf oils, with its sweet greenness.

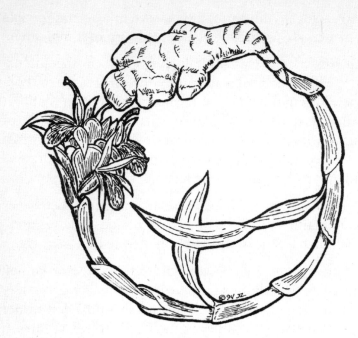

Ginger

Latin name: *Zingiber officinale.*

Botanical family: *Zingiberaceae.*

Origins: India, West Indies (particularly Jamaica), Africa, China, Philippines, Tahiti.

Part of plant used: Root.

Method of production: Distillation; yield one to three percent.

Evaporation rate: Middle to base.

Chemical constituents: Phellandrene, camphene, zingiberene, sesquiterpenoid alcohols, gingerol, gingerone, camphene.

Growing Habits

Ginger grows well in warm, humid, frost-free climates. The best ginger is said to come from Jamaica. It is a perennial, with a long stem three to four feet high and has round leaves six to twelve inches long and one to two inches wide. One type of stem bears leaves, and the other bears flowers, which are orchid-like and can be white, purple, or yellow. Hawaiian leis often have ginger lilies in addition to jasmine, carnation, and gardenia flowers. Propagation is by rhizome (or root) segments, this is the part of the plant valued for its medicinal qualities. The roots are dug up after the stems have withered, around January or February, then washed and dried. White ginger is ginger root which has been peeled. Black ginger is unpeeled. Green ginger is the fresh root, often used in cooking and ginger tea.

Plant lore

Ginger was one of the most prized of ancient remedies. The name ginger comes from a Latin word which derives from the Sansksrit, *grinavera,* which means "horn shaped body," referring to the shape of the roots. *Zingibar* was the ancient name used by the Greeks and Romans. Ginger is mentioned in the writings of Dioscorides and Hippocrates as having heating and digestive qualities. The Romans mainly used it in the culinary arts. It is native to Asia, and was grown in India and China, making its way to Europe via the spice route during the Middle Ages. It was important in Chinese medicine as a warming herb with a specific affinity for the lungs and intestines. The Spaniards introduced it to South America during the 16th century. In 1600, it was brought to England by a Lord Zouche, who was a great traveler and the owner of a famous botanical garden in London. During the Middle Ages it was a popular flavoring, and was used in almost every dish. In the *Doctrine of Signatures* it was felt to be of use to the digestive system because of its likeness to the convoluted intestines.

Therapeutic qualities

Carminative, stimulating, rubefacient, aperative, stomachic, antiseptic, tonic, febrifuge, analgesic.

Practical applications

- *Blending.* Ginger is nice with the citrus oils, and the woods and resins. A blend with eucalyptus or tea-tree might also be interesting, particularly for flu in the winter.

- *Digestive system.* Good for dyspepsia, flatulence, colic, gout, nausea, travel sickness, vomiting. Warms and stimulates stomach and intestines, helps make other formulas more acceptable by the digestive system (add a little fresh ginger, or ginger tincture to herbal infusions or other tinctures); also aids other oils to reach their target organs. Ginger tea for internal use: simmer one ounce of fresh ginger for ten minutes in one pint of water. Good for cramps, indigestion, nausea, and with honey and lemon for colds and flu.

- *Respiratory system.* Ginger stimulates the lungs to expel phlegm and also helps to stimulate the immune system. The Chinese consider it to be one of the prime lung remedies, with warming, dispersing, and drying qualities. Thus it is good for conditions where there is an excess of moisture, for example phlegm.

- *Excretory system.* Ginger is good for diarrhea.

- *Joint problems.* It is a wonderful addition to any blend for rheumatic pain, spinal or joint problems and muscular aches and pains, because of its warming and rubefacient qualities.

- *Reproductive system.* Helpful for stimulating delayed menstruation, and easing cramps. Also for the cold feeling of this time of the month, and promoting the flow if it seems sluggish.

Methods of use

I use ginger very sparingly, maybe three drops in one ounce of carrier oil, or as part of a blend.

- *Digestive system.* Tea, local massage over the abdomen.

- *Respiratory system.* Chest rub, ginger in the bath, hot ginger tea with lemon and honey, burners.

- *Excretory system.* Baths, local massage over the abdomen and kidneys.

- *Joints.* Local massage oil, hot compresses, baths.
- *Reproductive system.* Local massage, baths, compresses to abdomen.

Further notes

Ginger is one of my favorite oils. I find its warming qualities a wonderful addition to many blends, and it is not so harsh as black pepper, for example. As an exercise, compare the various "hot" oils, and see if you can discern a difference in their warming qualities. Be careful with it though, as it can quickly become highly irritating if you use too much. For internal use, the tea can be useful, particularly in winter.

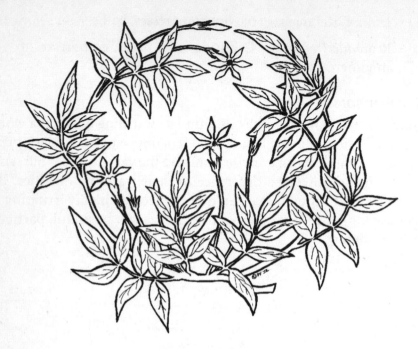

Jasmine

Latin names: *Jasminum officinalis, Jasminum grandiflorum.*

Botanical family: *Oleaceae.*

Origins: Iran, Kashmir, Northern India, Algeria, Morocco, France, China, Egypt, Italy, Turkey.

Part of plant used: Flowers.

Method of production: Enfleurage or solvent extraction.

Evaporation rate: Base.

Chemical constituents: Methyl anthranilate, indol, benzyl alcohol, benzyl acetate, linalol and linalyl acetate.

Growing habits

Jasmine is a vinelike climbing plant with white funnel-shaped flowers and small oval dark green leaves. It blooms from July to October, and is indigenous to the warm parts of the Eastern hemisphere. The flowers are gathered at night when the plant is at its most aromatic, and the flowers release essential oil for several days after harvesting. There are more than 200 species of jasmine, but the essential oil is taken from the two varieties named above.

Plant lore

The name jasmine comes from the Persian word *jasemin*, and the Arabic *ysmyn*. In the first century A.D., Dioscorides wrote that jasmine was used to perfume the air at banquets. To the Chinese, who use the variety *Jasminum sambac* to perfume their tea, it symbolized womanly sweetness. In India the oil was extracted by placing jasmine flowers amongst warm, hulled sesame seeds, which acquired the aroma of the flowers. This oil would be used to scent the hair and body. In medieval Christian art, jasmine was associated with the Virgin Mary. Dreaming of jasmine was supposed to portend good luck, especially in love, and in the language of flowers used in the Courtly Love of the Middle Ages, jasmine represented elegance.

Therapeutic qualities

Antidepressant, antiseptic, antispasmodic, aphrodisiac, galactagogic, parturient, sedative, tonic.

Practical applications

- *Blending.* Jasmine is so precious, it is a shame to blend it with anything else. Some people don't like the sweetness of it, and add bergamot to tone it down. Geranium also is a friend to jasmine.

- *Psychological effects.* Helps overcome lack of confidence, depression, and anxiety, instills optimism, fights indifference, postnatal depression. An aphrodisiac, restores sexual confidence.

- *Female problems.* Leucorrhea, promotes labor, analgesic in childbirth, promotes the flow of milk, helps with expulsion of placenta, helps fight frigidity.

- *Male sexual problems.* Helps with prostate problems, warms and strengthens male sexual organs.

- *Skin care.* Good for treating hot, dry, sensitive skin.

Methods of use

- *Psychological effects.* The prime method of use has to be massage, since it is on the emotional level that jasmine reigns supreme. It is too expensive to flush down the drain after a bath. It can also be used as a personal perfume by applying a drop to the wrists, heart, or behind the ears.

- *Female problems.* Jasmine is a wonderful massage oil in childbirth. It also can be inhaled or rubbed on the breasts in a very dilute form to promote milk flow when nursing.

- *Male sexual problems.* Can be used for a sexy massage or a personal perfume.

- *Skin care.* Lotions, facial oils, compresses.

Further notes

If rose is the queen of oils, jasmine is the king. The wonderful of aroma of jasmine is warm, sensual, reassuring, and instills a love of life when all seems too much to bear. Its beautiful scent makes this oil one of the best oils to use when psychological and emotional insecurities undermine one. It has great uplifting qualities, and a sweet, almost cloying quality that penetrates to the deepest recesses of the soul. One of the great essential oils.

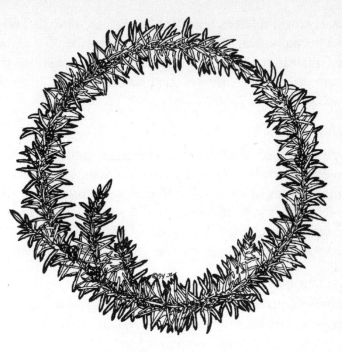

Juniper

Latin name: *Juniperus communis.*

Botanical family: *Cupressaceae.*

Origins: Canada, France, Italy, Morocco, Spain, Sweden, Yugoslavia.

Part of plant used: Berries, twigs, and wood. The best oil comes from the berries.

Method of production: Distillation; yield up to two percent.

Evaporation rate: Middle.

Chemical constituents: Essential oil containing borneol and isoborneol, cadinene, pinene, camphene, terpineol, terpenic alcohol, juniper camphor.

Growing habits

The juniper is a small evergreen tree with short, spiny leaves. It grows on chalk downs, heaths and moors, is four to twelve feet tall, and flowers from April to June. The berries are initially green, turning deep purple to black when ripe. The male plant has yellow flowers, the female green flowers. The berries that are distilled to extract the oil are produced by the female plant. Juniper is from the same family as cypress and pine.

Plant lore

In the past, juniper was considered a magical plant and was burned to ward off evil spirits, devils, and wild animals. It was used as a disinfectant in times of epidemics. In Germany it was used in Christmas celebrations to represent the "tree of life." In Christian mythology, it is mentioned as a symbol of protection. The Tibetans used juniper in religious ceremonies and for medical purposes.

Therapeutic qualities

Antidiabetic, antirheumatic, antitoxic, astringent, carminative, cicatrisant, depurative, diuretic, emmenagogic, nervine, rubefacient, stomachic, sudorific, tonic, excretory tract antiseptic.

Practical applications

- *Blending.* Juniper works well with bergamot, cypress, rosemary, frankincense, lavender, and sandalwood.

- *Excretory system.* Good for excretory tract infections and kidney stones. Can be irritating to the kidneys if used over a long period of time; alternate with sandalwood. Also a good diuretic and detoxifier. With frankincense, good for hemorrhoids. Do not use in cases of severe inflammation. Helps with toxicity and waste elimination.

- *Reproductive system.* Treats leuccorhea, ammenorhea, and dysmenorrhea.

- *Circulatory system.* Stimulates circulation; helps arteriosclerosis. A blood cleanser.

- *Nervous system.* Good for depletion, exhaustion, and lassitude. A psychic cleanser.

- *Skin care.* Dermatitis, eczema, acne, cellulite, toxicity, and congestion.

Methods of use

- *Excretory system.* Baths, massage, kidney compresses.

- *Reproductive system.* Douches, baths, abdomen massage, compresses.

- *Circulatory system.* Baths, massage.

- *Nervous system.* Baths, inhalations, burners, massage.

- *Skin care.* Baths, compresses, lotions.

Further notes

Patricia Davis considers juniper the classic oil for detoxification of mind and body. This is a good way to classify juniper, as a cleanser, with special affinity for the excretory system. For this reason, it is good for rheumatism and gout. Tisserand says:

> Considering its relatively mild toxicity, juniper is a remarkably effective and versatile remedy, with no contraindications. It should be used in conditions characterized by cold, fear, trembling, weakness, and languor.

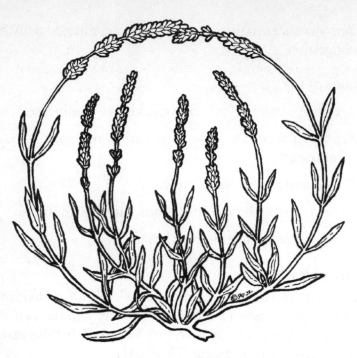

Lavender

Latin name: *Lavandula officinalis, Lavandula angustifolia,* or *Lavandula vera.*

Botanical family: *Lamiaceae* (mint family).

Origins: France, Spain, England, the former Soviet Union.

Part of plant used: Flowers.

Method of production: Distillation; yield 0.8 to 1.7 percent.

Evaporation rate: Middle.

Chemical constituents: Esters of linalyl and geranyl acetate, geraniol, linalol, cineol, d-borneol, limonene, l-pinene, carophyllene, butyric and valeric esters, coumarin, and over 100 additional components.

Growing habits

Lavender reaches a height of one to three feet and flowers from June to August. Flowers are mauve-purple. The best lavender grows above

3,000 feet elevation, in the sun, on well-drained sandy or chalky soil (although English lavender is well respected). The essential oil is actually produced and stored in the leaves; the oil glands are embedded amongst the tiny hairs which cover the plant. The flower buds are gathered for processing when in full bloom. There are about 20 different varieties of lavender grown; *Lavandula spica* is a more camphorous oil, which has been used for respiratory complaints. It is also used in soaps, household products, and perfume. *Lavandula hybrida* (a cross between *Lavandula angustifolia* and *Lavandula spica*) is an important oil; it has pushed down the production of true lavender and is often sold as lavender by unscrupulous dealers. *Lavandula spica* is not used much now, but *Lavandula hybrida* is grown all over the lower land in French alps (600 feet) with massive production of the essential oil.

Plant lore

It is believed that lavender was introduced to Britain and other Northern European countries by the Romans. The Latin word *lavare* means to wash, and lavender has been used in bathing for centuries. Lavender water is one of the oldest English perfumes; the commercial distillation is supposed to have begun in the early seventeenth century. It is said to be ruled by Mercury, this can be connected to its traditional application to the nervous system. An unromantic oil, it is also supposed to function traditionally as an anaphrodisiac. Sprinkling lavender on the head was supposed to aid in maintaining one's chastity. Lavender was said to be one of the herbs dedicated to Hecate, the goddess of witches and sorcerers, and her two daughters Medea and Circe.

Therapeutic qualities

Bactericide, sedative, analgesic, antispasmodic, anticonvulsive, antidepressive, antiseptic, cytophylactic, diuretic, insect repellent, antirheumatismal, parasitic, emmenagogic, antimigraine, chologogue, bechic, hypotensor, sudorific, increases alimentary canal secretions.

Practical applications

- *Blending.* Lavender is an oil which seems happier with company; it also seems to enhance the therapeutic qualities of other oils. I add it to a blend when I want to improve its aromatic quality, as lavender is a familiar and acceptable aroma to most people. It seems to blend well with other flower oils, citrus oils, and other plants of the *lamiaceae* family; for example, rosemary or marjoram.

- *Respiratory system.* Eases sinusitis, asthma, influenza, bronchitis, catarrh, whooping cough, throat infections, fevers.

- *Nervous system.* Helps migraine, nervous tension, stress, insomnia, fainting, hypertension. Generally soothing, sedating, and balancing for the nervous system.

- *Skin care.* Lavender is a classic remedy for burns and wounds, it is also used to treat abscesses, acne, dermatitis, eczema, pediculosis, and psoriasis.

- *Reproductive system.* Used for leucorrhoea, in childbirth to help even out contractions, and as an analgesic. It also helps to harmonize and regulate menstruation.

Methods of use

- *Respiratory system.* Inhalations, compresses, massages, chest rubs.

- *Nervous system.* Massage, baths, inhalations, burners.

- *Skin care.* Steaming, creams, lotions, oils, compresses.

- *Reproductive system.* Douches (dilute one percent), sitz baths, squatting inhalations, massage, baths, compresses.

Further notes

Lavender is one of the most well-loved and widely used of all aromatherapy oils. The keynote with lavender seems to be balance, and I particularly associate it with calming and soothing the nervous system. It can be considered the aromatherapy aspirin, because of its analgesic qualities. The other remarkable qualities of this oil are its antiseptic and cytophylactic properties, which means that it is a wonderful rejuvenating and healing oil for the skin. Its antibiotic qualities also make it useful for treating flu and other viral infections. Lavender is one of the few oils that is relatively safe for children, and very dilute lavender baths (one to two drops) will help a restless child to sleep.

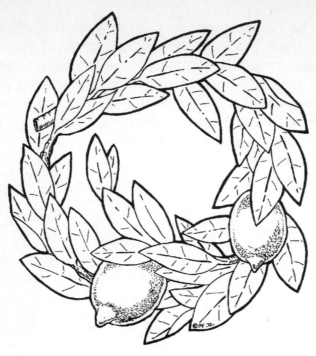

Lemon

Latin name: *Citrus limon.*

Botanical family: *Rutaceae.*

Origins: Argentina, Brazil, Cyprus, Portugal, Spain, the United States.

Part of plant used: Peel of the green fruit, which is richer in essential oils than when ripe.

Method of production: Expression; yield 0.1 to 0.3 percent.

Evaporation rate: Top.

Chemical constituents: Ninety-five percent terpenes (pinene, limonene, phellandrene, camphene, sesquiterpenes), linalol, acetates of linalyl and geranyl (esters), citral and citronella (aldehydes), camphor of lemon.

Growing habits

Lemon is cultivated in most subtropical and tropical countries. The lemon is one of the few trees that almost always has leaves, flowers, and fruit. It attains a height of 12 to 17 feet. The oil is in small pockets in the skin of the fruit, and is visible as small black dots.

Plant lore

The lemon is thought to have originated in India. It was introduced into Italy towards the end of the fifth century, and from there its cultivation spread throughout the Mediterranean region and to Spain and Portugal. It was first grown in California in 1887.

Therapeutic qualities

Lemon is a classic remedy with many uses. It is a bactericide, a strong antiseptic, activates the white corpuscles, is a febrifuge, a tonic for the nervous system, cardiotonic, alkalizing agent, antirheumatic, antigout, calmative, combats gastric acidity, diuretic, antiscorbutic, venous tonic, lowers hyperviscosity of the blood, hypotensive, depurative, rectifies mineral deficiencies, antianemic, aids pancreatic secretions, carminative, and vermifuge.

Practical applications

- *Blending.* Lemon blends well with other citrus oils, germanium, lavender, and neroli.

- *Immune system.* Helps fight infections of all kinds because of its action on the white corpuscles. Good for fighting head colds, sore throats, sinusitis, tonsillitis, inflammation of the mouth and gums, warts, and herpes. Its antibacterial and antiseptic actions are strong. It is good for lowering fevers, as it has a cooling action. It also purifies drinking water.

- *Circulatory system.* Has a blood-thinning and cleansing effect on the blood. It is good for arteriosclerosis, varicose veins, capillary fragility, hypertension, hemorrhage, nose bleeds, and chilblains.

- *Digestive system.* Despite its apparent acidity, lemon has an alkaline effect. It is good for any acidic condition, dyspepsia, vomiting, and pancreatic and hepatic inefficiency.

- *Antitoxicity.* Indicated for rheumatism, buildups of uric acid, arthritis, gout, and hepatic congestion.

- *Emotional problems.* Balances overly emotional states, brings feelings of light, clearness, and sharpness.

- *Skin care.* Lemon has a slight bleaching action on the skin, helps tighten stretched capillaries, is good for acne or infected skin conditions. It strengthens connective tissue, the acid mantle of the skin, and strengthens hair and nails. It is also claimed to tighten wrinkles.

Methods of use

- *Immune system.* Baths, burners, inhalations, massage. For warts, apply directly twice a day.

- *Circulatory system.* Baths, massage.

- *Digestive system.* Baths, compresses on the abdomen, local massage.

- *Antitoxicity.* Baths, local compresses, lemon juice (**not** lemon oil) in water, massage.

- *Psychological effects.* Baths, burners, inhalations, massage.

- *Skin care.* Facial lotions, lemon juice, massage, steaming.

Further notes

Valnet is the best source of information about lemon, and cites much evidence for its antiseptic properties. Writing about its antacid effect, he says, "Experiments have proved that prolonged use of lemons brings about within the organism the production of potassium carbonate which neutralizes excess acidity in the body fluids." He also notes that a few drops will kill 92 percent of all bacteria in oysters in 15 minutes. Lemon can be used internally very successfully in the form of lemon juice diluted in water.

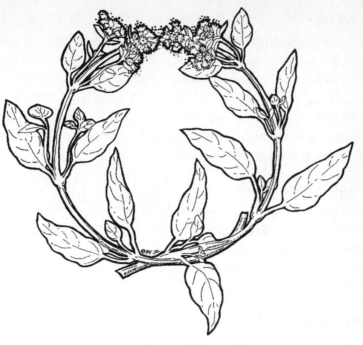

Marjoram

Latin name: Origanum majorana.

Botanical family: Lamiaceae.

Origin: France, England, Tasmania, Mediterranean area, Yugoslavia, Hungary, Iran.

Part of plant used: Flowering tops.

Method of production: Steam distillation.

Evaporation rate: Middle.

Chemical constituents: Terpenes, terpineol, sabines, carvacrol, borneol, camphor, origanol, pinene.

Growing habits

Marjoram is a perennial herb, growing one to three feet tall, with a hairy stem and flower stalks, small oval green leaves, and purple flowers at top of stems. Marjoram flowers June to October.

Plant lore

The name *origanum* means "joy of the mountain"; *majorana* means major, because it was once thought to bestow a long life span. The Greeks believed that the goddess Aphrodite first cultivated marjoram, and it was she who bestowed its wonderful fragrance. The Greeks wore wreaths of it as wedding flowers. It was also planted on graves because it was believed it would help the dead sleep in peace. No wonder it is so good for insomnia!

Therapeutic qualities

Marjoram is one of the most useful of the sedative oils in aromatherapy. It is also a good analgesic, anaphrodisiac, antiseptic, antispasmodic, carminative, cordial, carminative, digestive, emmenagogic, expectorant, hypotensor, laxative, nervine, sedative, tonic, and vasodilator.

Practical applications

- *Blending.* Marjoram blends well with lavender, rosemary, ylang-ylang, orange, and eucalyptus.

- *Circulatory system.* Its hypotensor, sedative, and vasodilator qualities make marjoram an excellent remedy for high blood pressure, palpitations, and anxiety symptoms. It helps dilate blood vessels and take the strain off the heart. It has a warming effect on the body, and is considered Yang.

- *Nervous system.* Its sedative properties make it a good general sedative; it also relaxes the nervous system. If abused, marjoram can have drug-like properties and can severely disorient you, so respect it. It is wonderful for migraines and insomnia.

- *Digestive system.* Marjoram increases peristalsis, so it is useful in cases of a cold and stagnant digestive and excretory system, and its antispasmodic properties help to ease griping pains in the stomach and intestines. It is also a good warming laxative.

- *Muscular system.* Marjoram is one of the most useful oils in general massage because of its ability to warm and relax the muscles and increase the local circulation. This helps to carry away waste products after exercise, and its analgesic quality helps to reduce pain. Its warmth and pain killing qualities are also comforting in arthritis and rheumatism. Its antispasmodic qualities make it wonderful for relaxing cramping or muscular spasms of any kind.

- *Reproductive system.* Marjoram makes a good warming emmenagogic, as well as a pain relieving antispasmodic for menstrual cramps. It also helps induce delayed periods. Because of its anaphrodisiac qualities, it will also help to balance excessive sexual impulses, and is useful when there is no immediate sexual outlet in someone's life.

- *Psychological effects.* Marjoram is warming and particularly comforting to the heart. Grief and loneliness are especially helped with marjoram; its warmth and penetrating aroma seems to sink to the depths of our pain and coldness, restoring our inner fire.

Methods of use

- *Circulatory system.* Massage, baths.

- *Nervous system.* Baths, massage, inhalation, diffusers, and burners, inhaling from a tissue or handkerchief, compresses for headaches, migraines.

- *Digestive system.* Taken as marjoram tea, compresses, massage over abdomen and intestinal area.

- *Muscular system.* Massage, compresses, baths.

- *Reproductive system.* Baths, massage, compresses, sitz baths.

- *Psychological effects.* Burners and diffusers, massage, baths.

Further notes

Marjoram is one of the most commonly used oils in aromatherapy, probably because of its applicability to most of the conditions related to stress. Most people, both men and women, like it. I use it instead of ginger or black pepper when I want to create inner warmth, but don't want to light a fire. Because it is a familiar scent to people, this itself makes them more comfortable.

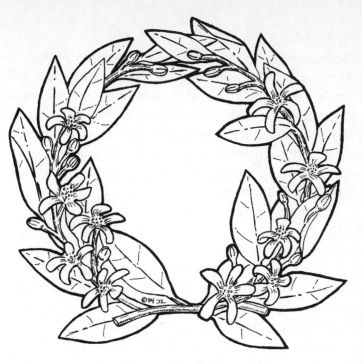

Neroli

Latin names: *Citrus aurantium* var. *amara* (bitter orange), *Citrus bigaradia.*

Botanical family: *Rutaceae.*

Origins: India, China, France, Italy, Sicily, Algeria, Iberian Peninsula, Mexico, California, South America, West Indies.

Part of plant used: Flowers.

Methods of production: Enfleurage, distillation, chemical solvents (often adulterated). One ton of flowers yields one kilogram of essential oil.

Evaporation rate: Middle to base.

Chemical constituents: Linalol, geraniol, nerol, benzoic, anthranilic and phenylacetic esters, traces of indole, jasmone, linalyl, geranyl, neryl acetate.

Growing habits

The plant is a small, evergreen tree which grows to a height of ten to twelve feet. It has a smooth, shiny trunk with grayish brown bark. The leaves are oval, three to four inches long, with oil vesicles. The flowers are white, the petals one half to one inch long, and are harvested in May. Three oils are produced from this tree. Neroli is from the flowers, petitgrain from the leaves and twigs, and bitter orange oil comes from the peel of the fruit. We also get orange flower water from distillation of the flowers.

Plant lore

The name for the plant derives from *citrus,* after the town of Citron in Judea, where it formerly flourished. *Aurantium* is from the Latin *aurum* for gold, referring to the color of the fruit. *Amara* is from the Latin *amarus,* which means bitter. The English word "orange" comes from the Sanskrit word *nagarange* and the Arabic *naranj.* The name *neroli* was adopted because the wife of the Prince of Nerola, in the 16th century, liked the perfume and made it very popular. The bitter orange tree is thought to have originated in southeast Asia or India. It is described in Chinese writings from 2200 B.C., but its use dates back much further. It was introduced to Europe by the Crusaders, and came to symbolize fecundity, as its tree bears fruit and blossoms at the same time. The use of orange flowers in the bridal bouquet and headdress was adopted in Europe around the seventeenth century. To the Chinese, the orange is a symbol of good luck and prosperity.

Therapeutic qualities

Antidepressive, antiseptic, antispasmodic, aphrodisiac.

Practical applications

- *Blending.* Neroli, lovely on its own, is also beautiful with rose and bergamot. A nice blend is neroli, petitgrain, and orange, which unites all of the oils from the same tree.

- *Nervous system and emotional balance.* Neroli is useful for shock, anxiety, and depression. It calms the spirit, is lightly hypnotic and slightly sedative, and is good for insomnia.

- *Circulatory system.* Diminishes cardiac contractions, palpitations, and angina.

- *Skin care.* Cytophilactic, rejuvenating. Good for dry, irritated, or sensitive skin.

- *Digestive and excretory system.* Relieves spasms in smooth muscle tissue, good for diarrhea, nervous dyspepsia.

Methods of use

- *Nervous system and emotional balance.* Baths, massage, as a personal perfume (an exquisite one, and a traditional use for neroli), burners, and diffusers.

- *Circulatory system.* Baths, massage, body oils, local compresses.

- *Skin care.* Skin care oils and lotions, compresses, orange flower water and infusions as toners, facial massage.

- *Digestive system.* Local massage and compresses.

Further notes

Neroli is one of the most beautiful and haunting of all essential oils. Its citrus qualities make it clear and clean, not as sickly as jasmine or ylang, although they are all flower oils. As an exercise it would be interesting to compare all of the flower oils, and see how they differ, depending on the type of plant, climate, and botanical family from which they come.

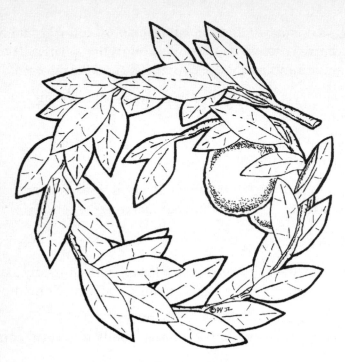

Orange

Latin names: *Citrus aurantium* var. *amara* (bitter), *Citrus aurantium* var. *dulcis* (sweet).

Botanical family: *Rutaceae.*

Origins: California, Israel, the Mediterranean, South America.

Part of plant used: Fruit peel.

Method of production: Expression.

Evaporation rate: Top.

Chemical constituents: Limonene (90 percent), citral, citronellal, geraniol, linalol (up to three percent), nerol, jasmone, anthranilic, benzioc and phenylacetic esters.

Growing habits

The orange is the fruit of an evergreen tree of the rue family. It grows best in warm tropical and subtropical regions all over the world, and requires good drainage and soil with a high content of organic matter. The aurantium variety is a small pyramid-shaped tree with oblong, shiny leaves and white flowers. The fruit is harvested by clipping the stems as close to the fruit as possible, and it must be handled carefully to avoid bruising the rind, which contains the precious essential oil sacs.

Plant lore
Originally a native of China and India, orange was not used medicinally in Europe until the late seventeenth century, because it was rare and expensive. The name comes from the Arabic *narandj,* which was transformed into the Spanish *naranja.* This fruit probably was the golden apple sought by Hercules in the Garden of the Hespeides.

Therapeutic qualities
Antidepressant, antispasmodic, digestive, mildly hypnotic and sedative, normalizes the peristaltic action of the intestines, stomachic.

Practical applications
- *Blending.* Orange goes well with spice oils, lavender and frankincense. It is particularly nice in a winter blend.

- *Digestive system.* Indigestion, dyspepsia, flatulence, gastric spasm.

- *Excretory system.* Diarrhea, constipation. Seems to balance the body fluids and help lymph to reach the tissues.

- *Psychological effects.* Warming, cheering, soothing. Calms nerves and corrects imbalance.

- *Skin care.* Softens the skin, plumps out tissues, hydrates, and brings warmth.

Methods of use
- *Digestive system.* Baths, massage over the abdomen.

- *Excretory system.* Baths, compresses, massage.

- *Psychological effects.* Baths, inhalations, massage.

- *Skin care.* Compresses, lotions, steaming.

Further notes

Little has been written about orange as an essential oil. We use three oils from the orange plant: neroli (bitter orange blossom), petitgrain (leaves and twigs), and orange itself. A nice idea for a beautiful blend is to reunite the three oils. Neroli and petitgrain share many qualities, except petitgrain has a woody, more earthy quality. Lemon and orange may be considered as complements. Lemon is more astringent, while orange is more open and expansive. Their respective shapes demonstrate this. Because orange can be irritating, it is wise to start with a one percent dilution, and to put no more than three drops in the bath.

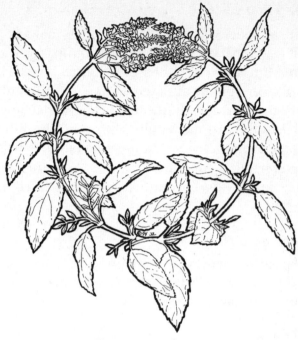

Peppermint

Latin name: Mentha piperata.

Botanical family: Labiatae.

Origins: Italy, the United States, Japan, Great Britain, Brazil, France.

Part of plant used: Leaves and flowering tops.

Method of production: Distillation; yield two to three percent.

Evaporation rate: Middle to top.

Chemical constituents: Terpenes (menthene, phellandrene, limonene), 30 to 70 percent menthol, ketone (menthone), and tannin.

Growing habits

Peppermint is a perennial that likes damp soil. It grows to about 20 inches, and flowers from June to August. The plants are gathered just before flowering. The best peppermint comes from England.

Plant lore

Discovered in a field in 1700 by John Rea, named peppermint because of its peppery smell. The mint family is said to derive its name from Minthe, the daughter of Cocytus. Minthe loved Pluto, when his wife Persephone discovered Pluto was unfaithful, in a jealous rage she transformed Minthe into the herb that bears her name. Mint was dedicated to the Virgin Mary, and the Romans placed bowls of peppermint leaves on banqueting tables to help curb their habit of overeating. Peppermint essence is one of the top selling essential oils in the world because it is so widely used in the flavoring industry.

Therapeutic qualities

Antigalactagogue, analgesic, antiphlogistic, antispasmodic, carminative, cephalic, cordial, febrifuge, hepatic, stimulant, sudorific, vasoconstrictor, emmenagogue, stomachic.

Practical applications

- *Blending.* Peppermint is very dominant, so use sparingly in the blend, or on its own. Blends well with benzoin and rosemary.

- *Digestive system.* Peppermint is one of the prime remedies for the digestive system, due to its antispasmodic, carminative, cordial, and stomachic qualities. It is indicated for indigestion, colic, flatulence, stomach pains, nausea, vomiting, sea or travel sickness, and diarrhea. It relieves internal toxicity and congestion, and has a strong effect on bile secretion due to its hepatic qualities. It is good for acute, short-term problems, while camomile can be used for a longer period of time. If using it for morning sickness, use the tea, and not in the first three months of pregnancy.

- *Nervous system.* One of the important qualities of peppermint is its cephalic effect, which it shares with basil and rosemary. It can be used in place of aspirin for headaches, and often helps with migraine, and clearing the liver congestion that can accompany this. There has always been controversy over whether peppermint is cooling or warming, as it feels cool, but is very stimulating to the circulation and nervous system. Its febrifuge qualities help bring fevers down.

- *Respiratory system.* Peppermint's cooling, antiseptic, expectorant qualities make it useful in lung and respiratory infection, and particularly sinusitis. It is good to use at the start of a cold or flu, to help arrest the chills.

- *Reproductive system.* Helps to relieve breast engorgement and tenderness associated with PMS. Can be used to help stop the flow of milk if this is desired.

Methods of use

- *Digestive system.* One drop in a glass of water, compresses, massage over the abdomen.

- *Nervous system.* Massage, compresses on forehead or back of neck for headaches, burners, inhalations.

- *Respiratory system.* Inhalations, burners, chest compresses, massage.

- *Reproductive system.* Compresses, massage.

Further notes

Peppermint should not be used in conjunction with homeopathic treatment, as it antidotes the remedies. Also do not to use it consistently in excessive amounts over a long period (more than a week if using solely peppermint), because it can lead to nervous disorder. Dilute to one percent for external use, and put no more than three drops in the bath. Use peppermint early in the day so as not to disturb your sleep patterns.

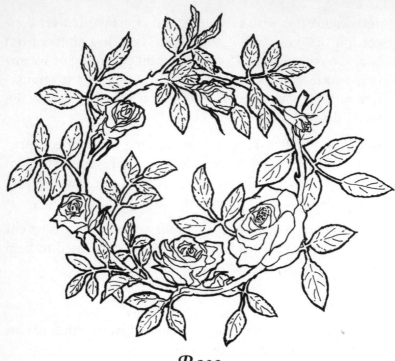

Rose

Latin names: *Rosa centifolia* (French, Moroccan rose), *Rosa damascena* (Turkish rose), *Rosa gallica.*

Botanical family: *Rosaceae.*

Origins: Bulgaria, Morocco, France, England, Turkey, the former Soviet Union, Syria, India.

Part of plant used: Flowers.

Method of production: Enfleurage, solvent extraction, and distillation, which yields rose otto. (This is the preferred oil for aromatherapeutic purposes. Absolute is reddish-orange, otto is pale yellow.) Yields one kilo of rose oil for 4000 kilos of flowers.

Evaporation rate: Middle to base.

Chemical constituents: Phenylethylic alcohols, geraniol, citronnellol, serol, acetates.

Growing habits

The rose is a hardy shrub growing up to four feet tall, with deep pinkish red, richly scented flowers and golden stamens followed by red rose hips. It has thorns and woody stems. It is propagated by planting cuttings in the autumn, and likes a sunny position and good loam. The roses used for the oil bloom for just 30 days, and are hand-picked in the morning during July and August. The harvest must be processed in 24 hours if it is to maintain its precious essential oil.

Plant lore

I could fill the remainder of the book with the story of the rose. It is one of the most precious and well-loved of all flowers, the queen herself. Most of the major spiritual traditions revere rose. The Christians believe it symbolizes the blood of Christ, for the Sufis it symbolizes the highest spiritual attainments, and a Muslim tradition credits the existence of rose to a drop of sweat which was left by Mohammed as he ascended to Heaven. It has always been the supreme symbol of love, and a bouquet of roses was found in the sarcophagus of King Tut, offered by his queen as a symbol of her devotion. The plant has been a symbol of love, beauty, perfection, and immortality. The thorns symbolize the pain of love and guilt, the withering blossom the ephemeral nature of beauty and youth. Different colored blooms symbolized different things: pink was simplicity or happy love, white was purity, yellow jealousy, and red was passion and sensual desire, shame, blood, and sacrifice. It is one of the oldest flowers in continual cultivation; fossilized traces of rose 35 million years old have been found in Montana, Colorado, and Oregon.

Therapeutic qualities

Antidepressant, anti-inflammatory, antiseptic, antispasmodic, aphrodisiac, astringent, emmenagogue, haemostatic, hepatic, laxative, purifying, sedative, splenetic, stomachic, uterine tonic.

Practical applications

- *Blending.* I think rose and lavender make a lovely blend, but in general I would suggest using it on its own to appreciate the beauty of this oil. One interesting blend a student created is rose and black pepper!

- *Psychological effects.* Eases grief, anger, jealousy, problems relating to the feminine, frigidity, inability to love, depression, loss of love. Aphrodisiac.

- *Reproductive system.* Rose is the supreme women's remedy. It has a tonic action on the uterus, is a gentle emmenagogue, helps regulate menstruation, and can help in adjusting to menopause. It helps with postnatal depression, and restores a woman's love of her femininity.

- *Skin care.* Rose is good for dry, aging, and sensitive skin. Rosewater is a good gentle skin tonic. Its astringent properties help mend broken capillaries. It is one of the most antiseptic, yet least toxic, oils.

- *Hepatic system.* Rose is specific to the liver, helps promote the flow of bile, and helps combat the effects of alcohol.

- *Circulatory system.* Promotes circulation, cleanses blood, and relieves cardiac congestion. It tones the capillaries, and has a gentle decongesting, rather than stimulating, action.

Methods of use

- *Psychological effects.* Massage, inhalations, personal perfumes. A little too expensive to burn.

- *Reproductive system.* General or local massage, compresses, sitz baths.

- *Skin care.* Rose water, massage, lotions, compresses.

- *Hepatic system.* Local massage, compresses.

- *Circulatory system.* Massage.

Further notes

Despite its gentle manner, rose is a very powerful oil, particularly on the emotional plane, so be prepared for emotional release when using this oil. It is the supreme remedy for women and speaks to them with real understanding and depth. If I could choose only one oil to use for the rest of my life it would have to be rose. Although it is expensive and precious, it is worth every penny. Please do not be tempted to substitute a synthetic rose scent for the real thing.

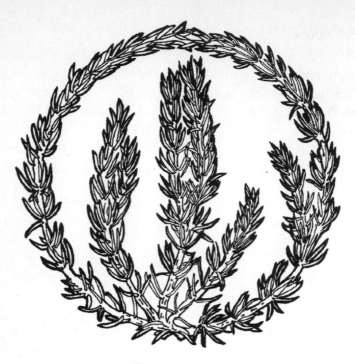

Rosemary

Latin name: *Rosmarinus officinalis.*

Botanical family: *Lamiaceae* (mint family).

Origins: The Mediterranean, Spain, S. France, Italy, Tunisia.

Part of plant used: Flowering tops and twigs.

Method of production: Distillation; yield 1.5 percent.

Evaporation rate: Middle.

Chemical constituents: Pinene, camphene, cineol, borneols (15 percent), camphors, resin, a bitter principal, saponin.

Growing habits

Rosemary grows from sea level up to 2000 feet, and prefers rocky, sunny slopes, or dry, sandy soil. It is a favorite plant for bees, and the plant flowers from May to July. It has pale to medium blue flowers, and grows up to six feet tall. Rosemary oil is often adulterated with turpentine, sage, or spike oils. The essential oil is stored in goblet-shaped cells just below the leaf surface.

Plant lore

The legend is that originally the flowers were white, but they turned blue when the Virgin Mary hung her blue cloak over a rosemary bush. It was also believed that it grew to the height of Christ in 33 years, and after that got thicker, but not taller. For the Greeks and Romans, rosemary symbolized love and death, and these associations stayed with the plant through the ages. Greek students wore garlands of rosemary to enhance their memories when studying for exams. The first known distillation of rosemary essential oil was by Raymond Tully in 1330.

Therapeutic qualities

Astringent, adrenal cortex stimulant, analgesic, antiseptic, antidiarrhea, general stimulant, cardiac tonic, hypertensive, carminative, antirheumatic, antineuralgic, antigout, chologogue, emmenagogue, cerebral stimulant, sudorific, arasiticide, cicatrisant, cephalic, hepatic, nervine, vulnary.

Practical applications

- *Blending.* Generally, rosemary blends well with other lamiaceaes, basil, frankincense, and cedarwood. It has a strong aroma, so use it in moderation, and whenever you want to add stimulating qualities to a blend.

- *Circulatory system.* Combats arteriosclerosis, high cholesterol, hypotension, hepatic disorders, cirrhosis, gall stones, gout, bile secretions.

- *Nervous system.* General stimulant, fainting, headache, mental fatigue.

- *Digestive system.* Diarrhea, tonic to the digestion. Hepatic stimulant and detoxifier.

- *Reproductive system.* Emmenogogue.
- *Additional uses.* Overworked muscles, circulatory stimulant, arthritis and rheumatism, and scalp disinfectant and tonic.

Methods of use

- *Circulatory system.* Baths, massage.
- *Hepatic system.* Local applications, baths, massage.
- *Nervous system.* Inhalations, massage, baths.
- *Digestive system.* Local application, baths, massage, compresses.
- *Reproductive system.* Massage, sitz baths, compresses, local applications.
- *Muscles and joints.* Local massage, baths, compresses. Additional uses include scalp massage and warm oil treatments.

Further notes

Rosemary should be thought of as the complement to lavender. Where lavender is calming, rosemary is stimulating. Its main field of action seems to be in the circulatory and nervous systems. It also targets the liver, and its piercing bactericidal qualities make it a good respiratory remedy. This is an oil to be respected, as it can be toxic in large doses, and you should keep it away from anyone who has a history of epilepsy. In skin care it can be very useful for congested skin. One of the most famous aromatic waters, Hungary Water, was based on this plant. Generally, rosemary pierces, stimulates, and sharpens all it comes in contact with.

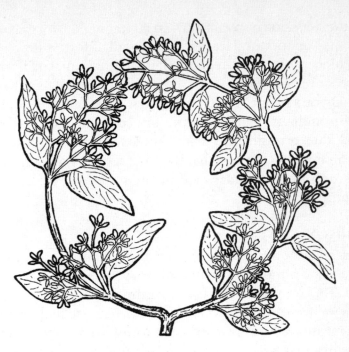

Sandalwood

Latin name: Santalum album.

Botanical family: Santalaceae.

Origins: India, E. Indian Islands, Australia (*Sandelwood spicatum*).

Part of plant used: Heartwood.

Method of production: Distillation; yield 3.5 percent.

Evaporation rate: Base.

Chemical constituents: Eighty percent alcohols: santalol, fusanol, santalic acid, terasantalic acid, and carbides.

Growing habits

The sandalwood tree has a very interesting story. Although it is capable of photosynthesis, it is a parasite, and parasitizes the roots of other trees to obtain nitrogen and phosphorous. This eventually kills the host, which might be such trees as teak, clove, bamboo, or guava.

It grows very slowly, reaching 20 to 30 feet high, with grayish brown bark and smooth oval leaves. It has small, odorless flowers of various colors: violet, pink, red, or yellow. The essential oil is found only in trees over 25 years old, so the trees are harvested at between 30 and 60 years of age. Once the tree has been felled, it is allowed to remain on the ground until white ants consume the outer white sapwood, thus exposing the yellow heartwood. So much sandalwood was cut down in the past that the Indian government now controls the production of sandalwood oil, and the trees are cultivated for this purpose.

Plant lore

The sandalwood tree has a long tradition of use. It has a very hard, dense wood almost the texture of ivory when it is carved and polished. This accounts for its use in creating fine carvings, such as statues, jewel boxes, and the carved ribs for Chinese folding fans which were introduced from Japan in the Ming dynasty. In India, important entryways were carved in sandalwood because of its resistance to termites and lovely scent, and sandalwood and other spices were used to cover the odor of cremations. The third-eye dot between the eyes was made with sandalwood paste, to symbolize the gaze within. Here we see its links with incense, perfume, and meditation; its soft scent was thought to induce calmness and serenity. In perfumery, sandalwood is one of the classic base notes, and is the base for many green and woody perfumes. The Sanskrit word is *chandana*, to shine; the English is derived from the Persian *sandul*, or useful, and *album* means white or light. Sandalwood has been used for thousands of years in the East, and in Ayurvedic medicine as a cooling remedy. It is mentioned in the *Mahabharata*, in Ruamyana epic poems of India, and in the *Nirukta*, written during the fifth century B.C.

Therapeutic qualities

Antidepressant, antiseptic, antispasmodic, astringent, aphrodisiac, bactericidal, carminative, expectorant, sedative, tonic.

Practical applications

- *Blending.* Lovely blended with rose, jasmine, bergamot, and other citrus oils, also resins like benzoin and myrrh. As a base note, is a good fixative for other oils, and if used sparingly adds weight without dominating the blend.

- *Respiratory system.* Bronchitis, inflammations, and infections of the lungs with fever, chronic and subacute inflammations of the mucous membranes, dry and persistent coughs, sore throats, laryngitis, tuberculosis.

- *Excretory system.* Diarrhea, cystitis.

- *Skin care.* Dry and irritated skin, mildly astringent, and soothing for acne.

- *Reproductive system.* Gonorrhea, aphrodisiac, genital discharges in male and female.

- *Nervous system.* Depression, insomnia, nervous tension.

Methods of use

- *Respiratory system.* Inhalations, chest rubs/compress, baths.

- *Eliminatory system.* Baths, massage, sitz baths.

- *Skin care.* Facial oil or lotion, compresses, facial steam.

- *Reproductive system.* Baths, massage, compresses.

- *Nervous system.* Diffusers and burners, massage, baths.

Further notes

In traditional medicine, sandalwood is of a cool, dry nature; this shows its anti-inflammatory and damp-arresting qualities. It can be seen as the opposite of ginger, which is hot and dry. It has some soothing qualities, like its ability to soothe dry, dehydrated skin, so maybe sandalwood also has the ability to balance moisture in some way. It is one of the deepest acting, most clinging oils, and despite its soft, mellow aroma, is powerful in its effect. A nice oil for men.

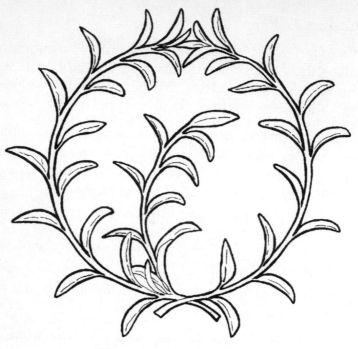

Tea-tree or Ti-tree

Latin name: *Melaleuca alternifolia.*

Botanical family: *Myrtaceae.*

Origin: Australia.

Part of plant used: Leaves.

Method of production: Distillation.

Evaporation rate: Middle.

Chemical constituents: Terpineol, alcohols, monoterpenes.

Growing habits

Tea-trees were originally found only in a small swampy area along the northern coast of New South Wales. They have a long trunk and branches, with the leaves on the top, and are so prolific that if pruned to within two feet of the ground, the tree will again have thick foliage within 18 months. Recently the demand for tea-tree oil has sky-rocketed, and plantations are now being created to insure supply.

Plant lore

Tea-tree is an old aboriginal remedy. The Bundjaling used crushed leaves as a poultice for infected wounds and skin problems. It was named tea-tree when Captain Cook and his sailors brewed the leaves as a change from their ordinary tea, and found it to be a spicy, pleasant beverage. It is one of the most scientifically researched essential oils, and in 1925 A.R. Penfold, an Australian government chemist, was the first to publish the fact that tea-tree oil is twelve times stronger than phenol. In 1930, a paper in the *Medical Journal of Australia* commented on its nontoxicity and its effectiveness as a germicidal agent. In 1937 it was noted that pus, blood, or other organic fluids actually increase the antiseptic power of the oil by ten to twelve percent. After World War II, interest in the oil declined with the widespread use of antibiotics, but since then, tea-tree oil has been studied by many people, and you could say it has become the miracle cure of the nineties, particularly with so much concern about immune enhancement and the strange viruses that are around.

Therapeutic qualities

Antibiotic, antiseptic, antiviral, bactericidal, fungicidal, immunostimulant, cardiac tonic, sudorific.

Practical applications

- *Blending.* Tea-tree tends to dominate a blend. A powerful therapeutic blend is tea-tree and clove or eucalyptus, since they are in the same family. Tea-tree and lavender is pleasant. It also blends well with citrus oils such as orange or lemon.

- *Reproductive system.* Trichomonal vaginitis, other vaginal infections, leucchorea.

- *Excretory system.* Chronic cystitis, urinary infections.

- *Skin care.* Acne, burns, diaper rash, ulcers, wounds, psorasis.

- *Respiratory system.* Colds, flus, throat, bronchial, sinus infections.

- *Periodontal care.* Infected gums, mouth ulcers.

- *Immune system.* French physicians are doing research using tea-tree for AIDS treatment, as well as all of the above, and also use it to strengthen the immune system before surgery. Viral infections: Herpes, influenza, warts, Epstein-Barr, glandular fever, shingles, chicken pox (herpes zoster). Fungal infections: Athlete's foot, ringworm, fungal infections under toenails. Yeast imbalance. Candida albicans, thrush.

Methods of use

- *Reproductive system.* Tampon soaked in a dilute (one percent) solution of tea-tree, douches, baths, vaginal pessaries.

- *Excretory system.* Sitz baths, compresses, baths, local cream.

- *Skin care.* Lotions, massage, steaming, compresses, baths.

- *Respiratory/sinus system.* Facial massage oil, inhalations, chest rubs, chest compresses, baths.

- *Periodontal care.* Mouthwashes, diluted in carrier oil and rubbed on the gums.

- *Immune system.* Massage (regular and lymphatic), baths, apply to lymph glands, burners. Viral infections. Baths, regular massages, burners, inhalations. Fungal infections. Foot bath, as a skin lotion, in the bath, compresses. Yeast imbalances. Massage oil, bath, local sitz bath, lotions.

Further notes

After lavender, tea-tree is one of the most useful oils in the aromatherapist's repertoire. Eucalyptus is specific to the lungs and respiratory system, while tea-tree has the unique feature of acting against all three categories of infectious organisms: bacteria, fungi, and viruses. It is the most powerful immune-stimulant we have. There is much research available on this oil now; one of the reasons for this is the French interest in replacing antibiotics with essential oils. Gynecological applications are also an area of interest for the use of tea-tree, particularly against candida. It is interesting that these problems arise from disharmony in systems that are usually self-regulating.

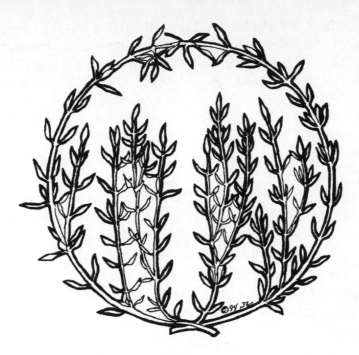

Thyme

Latin name: *Thymus vulgaris. Thymus zygis* and *Thymus citriodora* are also distilled.

Botanical family: *Lamiaceae.*

Origin: Morocco, Spain, France, Greece, Mediterranean region.

Part of plant used: Leaves and twigs.

Method of production: Distillation; yield 1.5 to 2.5 percent.

Evaporation rate: Middle.

Chemical constituents: Thymol, carvacrol (up to 60 percent), terpinene, cymene, borneol, linalol. Thyme is a good example of an oil whose chemical constituents change with the environment in which it is grown. Several chemotypes are used in clinical aromatherapy, and the properties of the chemotypes are quite distinct. The thymol chemotype is strong, bactericidal, immuno-stimulant and antiseptic. It can also be extremely irritating, and toxic in high doses. The linalol chemotype (referred to as sweet thyme) is gentle, nonirritating, and can be used with children. It is bactericidal, toning, and diuretic. The thujanol-4 chemotype is antiviral in its action. Red thyme is the first distillate, white thyme oil has been redistilled or rectified.

Growing habits

Thyme likes warmth and light. It will grow at both high and low altitudes. The thyme grown at higher altitudes is of the cooler, more soothing type, while that grown in lower, warmer environments displays more aggressive, irritating tendencies. *Thymus vulgaris,* or common thyme, is a cultivated form of *thymus serpyllum,* wild thyme, or "mother of thyme." It is a perennial plant with a woody root, hard stems, dark green tiny leaves, and a small lilac flower. It flowers from May to September, and grows 12 to 18 inches high. It attracts bees, and is often planted near hives.

Plant lore

The name thyme comes from the Greek word *thymus,* to perfume or fumigate, and because of its strong, invigorating smell it was used in the temples as incense. It has a long history of use by all of the early civilizations as a medicinal plant, and Hippocrates and Dioscorides described its properties. Of course, we all know it as a culinary herb. Infusions of thyme are considered to be a good substitute for coffee and tea because of its stimulating and tonic properties. In medieval times it was a symbol of courage, and knights parted for the Crusades with scarves embroidered with a sprig of thyme. Thyme tea was said to prevent nightmares, and to enable one to see fairies and nymphs. By the sixteenth century, it was cultivated in England and sold in London markets.

Therapeutic qualities

Stimulant, nerve tonic, hypotensive, antispasmodic, expectorant, antiseptic, stimulates leucocytosis, emmenagogue, sudorific, vermifuge, bactericide, antivenomous, antiputrifactive, parasiticide.

Practical applications

- *Blending.* Sweet thyme blends well with lemon, lavender, rosemary, orange, sweet thyme, and tea-tree.

- *Respiratory system.* Emphysema, mycosis, bronchitis, flu originating from chill, colds, expectorant.

- *Immune system.* Encourages leucocytosis, adrenal stimulant, general tonic for fatigue, convalescence, lack of *chi.* A good blend for increasing leucocytosis is thyme, lemon, lavender, and bergamot.

- *Circulatory system.* Raises low blood pressure, stimulates circulation, warmth, increases metabolism, promotes purification, cleansing of blood, stimulates spleen.

- *Nervous system.* Stimulates nervous system, mental clarity, sharpness.

- *Skin care.* Red thyme can be a skin irritant, use carefully; cicatrisant (helps in healing of difficult wounds and abrasions), increases circulation, clears congested skin, antiseptic, acne, stimulates glands, scalp problems.

- *Excretory system.* Stimulates kidneys, helps with excretion, fights infections, antiseptic.

- *Periodontal care.* Dilution of less than 0.10 percent is effective against bacteria which cause most mouth and gum infections.

- *Reproductive system.* Red thyme is a strong emmenagogue, and should not be used at all by pregnant women. I know of someone who was taking the contraceptive pill, and just smelling thyme induced a period.

Methods of use

- *Respiratory system.* Inhalations, baths, chest compresses, chest rubs, burners.

- *Immune system.* Baths, massage, inhalations, burners (also see tea-tree).

- *Circulatory system.* Massage, baths.

- *Nervous system.* Inhalations, baths, massages, apply along spine.

- *Skin care.* Lotions, facial oils, baths, compresses.

- *Excretory system.* Abdominal massage, compresses and massage to kidney area, baths, application of external lotion.

- *Periodontal care.* As a gargle. One drop in a cup of warm water.

- *Reproductive system.* Baths, massage, abdomen compress.

Further notes

Red thyme is one of the most powerful oils available and should be respected. It must be used in very dilute quantities; always start with a one percent dilution and work your way up. It is largely composed of phenols, which can be the most irritating oils. When tested against other oils for antiseptic, bactericidal, and antigenetic (antigerm) oils, thyme tops the list. Be careful about overuse—excessive doses can lead to vomiting, depression, coldness, and exhaustion.

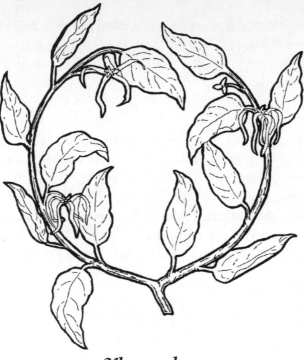

Ylang-ylang

Latin name: *Canaga odorata.*

Botanical family: *Annonaceae.*

Origins: Reunion, Comoro Islands, Madagascar, Java, Sumatra, Philippines, Malaysia, Seychelles, Tahiti, India.

Part of plant used: Flowers.

Method of production: Distillation. Five grades of oil are produced; the first distillate is premium or "extra," the last oil is canaga oil.

Evaporation rate: Middle to base.

Chemical constituents: Eugenol, geraniol, linalol, sasfrol, ylangol, terpenes, pinene, benzoate of benzyl, acetic, benzoic, formic, salicylic and valeric acids.

Growing habits
The canaga tree grows to about 60 feet high, does best at high eleva-

tions with dry soil, shade, spring rain, and blossoms all year. It has dark green oval leaves. The best flowers for oil are the yellow ones, although it also has pink and mauve ones. The best flowers for oil production are picked in May and June.

Plant lore

The ylang-ylang flower was discovered on Ceram in the Indonesian archipelago by Captain D'Etchevery in 1770; use of its scent did not take place until a German, Albertino Schwenger, was shipwrecked in the Philippines. He tried to distill it, having fallen in love with the perfume. Another German L. Steck, an apothecary, successfully cultivated and distilled ylang-ylang and exhibited it at the Paris World Exhibition in 1878. In 1893 it was introduced to Reunion.

Therapeutic qualities

Hypotensive, aphrodisiac, antidepressive, sedative, euphoric, antiseptic.

Practical applications

- *Blending.* I like ylang-ylang with the citrus oils: lemon, bergamot, and orange. Lime might be interesting. Clove would add fire. Sandalwood would make it deeper and grounded—very sexy indeed. Ylang-ylang seems to be a mixture of fire and water.

- *Nervous system and psychological effects.* Anxiety, anger, insomnia, nervous tension, depression, impotence, frigidity through fear and nervousness, shock, hyperpnea.

- *Circulatory system.* Palpitations, high blood pressure.

- *Excretory system.* Chronic diarrhea.

- *Skin care.* Oily skin, tonic effect on scalp.

Methods of use

- *Nervous system and psychological effects.* Baths, burners, massage.

- *Circulatory system.* Massage, baths.

- *Excretory system.* Local massage.

- *Skin care.* Compresses, facial oil or lotion.

Further notes

Many people find ylang-ylang an extremely effective aphrodisiac, while others find it nauseatingly sweet. It is widely used in perfumery, and has been called the poor man's jasmine because of its exotic, heavy aroma. It certainly has an euphoric quality.

Useful Addresses

For aromatherapy tuition and essential oils

Ann Berwick Aromatherapy
P.O. Box 4996
Boulder, CO 80306

Associations

The National Association for Holistic Aromatherapy
P.O. Box 17622
Boulder, CO 80308-7622

The International Society of Professional Aromatherapists
c/o Hinkley and District Hospital and Health Center
The Annex, Mount Road
Hinkley
Leics LE10 1AG England   Tel: 0455-637987

The International Federation of Aromatherapists
46 Dalkeith Road
Dulwich
London SE21 8LS England

Publications

Scentsitivity
Membership newsletter of the National Association for
Holistic Aromatherapy

The International Journal of Aromatherapy
P.O. Box 746
Hove, E. Sussex BN3 3XA England

Aromatherapy Quarterly
5 Raneleigh Avenue
London SW13 OBY England

Bibliography

Culpeper, N. *Culpeper's Complete Herbal.* London, England: W. Foulsham & Co.

Cunningham, S. *Magical Aromatherapy.* St. Paul, Minnesota: Llewellyn Publications, 1989.

Davis, P. *Aromatherapy: An A-Z.* Saffron Walden, England: C. W. Daniel, 1988.

Francômme, P. *Phytoguide No. 1: Aromatherapy, Advanced Therapy for Infectious Illnesses.* La Courtete, France: International Phytomedical Foundation, 1985.

Gumbel, G. *Principles of Holistic Skin Therapy with Herbal Essences.* Heidelberg, Germany: Haug, 1986.

Hoffman, D. *The Holistic Herbal.* Forris, Scotland: The Findham Press, 1983.

Holy Bible, Exodus 30, Verse 22.

Juneman, M. *Enchanting Scents.* Wilmot, Wisconsin: Lotus Press, 1988.

Karagulla, S. and D. van Gelder Kunz. *The Chakras and the Human Energy Fields.* Wheaton, Illinois: Quest Books, Theosophical Publishing House, 1989.

Maury, M. *Marguerite Maury's Guide to Aromatherapy: The Secret of Life and Youth.* Saffron Walden, England: C. W. Daniel, 1989.

Morris, E. *Fragrance.* Greenwich, Connecticut: E. T. Morris & Co., 1984.

Price, S. *Practical Aromatherapy: How to Use Essential Oils to Restore Vitality.* Wellingborough, England: Thorsons, 1987.

Price, S. *Aromatherapy for Common Ailments.* New York: Fireside, 1991.

Rowett, H. *Basic Anatomy and Physiology.* London: John Murray, 1959.

Tisserand, R. *To Heal and Tend the Body.* Wilmot, Wisconsin: Lotus Press, 1988.

Tisserand, R. *The Art of Aromatherapy.* Saffron Walden, England: C. W. Daniel, 1977.

Valnet, J. *The Practice of Aromatherapy.* Saffron Walden, England: C. W. Daniel, 1980.

Worwood, V. *Aromantics.* London: Pan Books, 1987.

Index

A

acids, 20

adrenal cortex, 111, 114, 119, 137, 164-5, 201

adulteration, 18

air disinfectant, 40, 174

air freshener, 40

alchemy, 6

alcohols, 14, 20, 135

aldehydes, 20, 26, 135

allergies, 18, 74, 81, 102

almond oil, 94,107

analgesic, 88, 140, 143-4, 154, 164, 167, 171, 177-9, 184-5, 194, 201

annonaceae, 213

antiallergic, 143

antibacterial, 181

antibiotic, 21, 179, 207

anticonvulsive, 143, 147, 177

antidepressant, 24, 137, 140, 144, 164-5, 171, 191, 197

antidiabetic, 164-5, 174

antifungal, 103, 105, 135

antigalactagogic, 147

anti-inflammatory, 20, 75, 78-9, 144, 164, 197, 205

antineuralgic, 155, 201

antiphlogistic, 135, 143, 145, 194

antirheumatic, 147, 151, 155, 174, 181, 201

antiseptic, 7, 19-21, 38, 40, 57, 73, 78, 81, 134, 137, 140, 143-4, 147, 154-5, 158-159,161, 164-5, 167, 171, 174, 177, 179, 181-2, 184, 188, 195, 197-8, 201, 207, 209-12, 214

antispasmodic, 58, 137-8, 140, 143-4, 147-8, 151, 154, 158, 171, 177, 184-5, 188, 191, 194, 197, 210

antitoxic, 158, 174

antitussive, 58

antiviral, 57, 103-4, 114, 135, 141, 154,

Stay in Touch

On the following pages you will find some of the books now available on related subjects. Your book dealer stocks most of these and will stock new Llewellyn titles as they become available.

To obtain our full catalog, to keep informed about new titles as they are released, and to benefit from informative articles and helpful news, you are invited to write for our bimonthly news magazine/catalog, *Llewellyn's New Worlds of Mind and Spirit*. A sample copy is free, and it will continue coming to you at no cost as long as you are an active mail customer. Or you may subscribe for just $10.⁰⁰ in the U.S.A. and Canada ($20.⁰⁰ overseas, first class mail). Many bookstores also have *New Worlds* available to their customers. Ask for it.

Llewellyn's New Worlds of Mind and Spirit
P.O. Box 64383-678, St. Paul, MN 55164-0383, U.S.A.

To Order Books and Tapes

If your book dealer does not have the books described, you may order them directly from the publisher by sending the full price in U.S. funds, plus $3.⁰⁰ for postage and handling for orders under $10.⁰⁰; $4.⁰⁰ for orders over $10.⁰⁰. There are no postage and handling charges for orders over $50.⁰⁰. Postage and handling rates are subject to change. We ship UPS whenever possible. Delivery guaranteed. Provide your street address as UPS does not deliver to P.O. Boxes. UPS to Canada requires a $50.⁰⁰ minimum order. Allow 4-6 weeks for delivery. Orders outside the U.S.A. and Canada: Airmail—add retail price of book; add $5.⁰⁰ for each nonbook item (tapes, etc.); add $1.⁰⁰ per item for surface mail.

For Group Study and Purchase

Because there is a great deal of interest in group discussion and study of the subject matter of this book, we offer a special quantity price to group leaders or agents. Our Special Quantity Price for a minimum order of five copies of *Holistic Aromatherapy* is $38.⁸⁵ cash-with-order. This price includes postage and handling within the United States. Minnesota residents must add 6.5% sales tax. For additional quantities, please order in multiples of five. For Canadian and foreign orders, add postage and handling charges as above. Credit card (VISA, MasterCard, American Express) orders are accepted. Charge card orders only ($15.⁰⁰ minimum order) may be phoned in free within the U.S.A. or Canada by dialing 1-800-THE-MOON. For customer service, call 1-612-291-1970. Mail orders to:

Llewellyn Publications
P.O. Box 64383-678, St. Paul, MN 55164-0383, U.S.A.

MAGICAL AROMATHERAPY
The Power of Scent
by Scott Cunningham

Scent magic has a rich, colorful history. Today, in the shadow of the next century, there is much we can learn from the simple plants that grace our planet. Most have been used for countless centuries. The energies still vibrate within their aromas.

Scott Cunningham has now combined the current knowledge of the physiological and psychological effects of natural fragrances with the ancient art of magical perfumery. In writing this book, he drew on extensive experimentation and observation, research into 4,000 years of written records, and the wisdom of respected aromatherapy practitioners. *Magical Aromatherapy* contains a wealth of practical tables of aromas of the seasons, days of the week, the planets, and zodiac; use of essential oils with crystals; synthetic and genuine oils and hazardous essential oils. It also contains a handy appendix of aromatherapy organizations and distributors of essential oils and dried plant products.

0-87542-129-6, 224 pgs., mass market, illus.   **$3.95**

MAGICAL HERBALISM
The Secret Craft of the Wise
by Scott Cunningham

Certain plants are prized for the special range of energies they possess. *Magical Herbalism* unites the powers of plants and man to produce, and direct, change in accord with human will and desire.

It's Magic as old as our knowledge of plants, an art that anyone can learn and practice, and once again enjoy as we look to the Earth to rediscover our roots and make inner connections with Nature.

This is the Magic of Enchantment, of word and gesture to shape the images of mind and channel the energies of the herbs. It is a Magic for everyone—the herbs are easily and readily obtained, the tools are familiar or easily made, and the technology is of home and garden. This book includes step-by-step guidance to the preparation of herbs and to their compounding in incense and oils, sachets and amulets, simples and infusions, with simple rituals and spells for every purpose.

0-87542-120-2, 260 pgs., 5 1/4 x 8, illus., softcover   **$7.95**

JUDE'S HERBAL HOME REMEDIES
Natural Health, Beauty & Home-Care Secrets
by Jude C. Williams, M.H.

There's a pharmacy in your spice cabinet! Every day we encounter problems—headaches, dandruff, insomnia, colds, burns, etc.—that can be easily remedied using common herbs. *Jude's Herbal Home Remedies* is a simple guide to self care that will benefit beginning to experienced herbalists with a wealth of practical advice.

Discover how cayenne pepper promotes hair growth, why cranberry juice is a good treatment for asthma attacks, how to make a potent juice to flush out fat, how to make your own deodorants and perfumes, what herbs will get fleas off your pet, how to keep cut flowers fresh longer…the remedies and hints go on and on!

This book gives you instructions for teas, salves, tinctures, tonics, poultices, along with addresses for obtaining the herbs. Dangerous and controversial herbs are also discussed. Discover from a Master Herbalist more than 800 ways to a simpler, more natural way of life.
0-87542-869-X, 240 pgs., 6 x 9, illus., softcover $9.⁹⁵

HEALING HERBS & HEALTH FOODS OF THE ZODIAC
by Ada Muir, Introduction by Jude C. Williams, M.H.

There was a time when every doctor was also an astrologer, for a knowledge of astrology was considered essential for diagnosing and curing an illness. *Healing Herbs and Health Foods of the Zodiac* reclaims that ancient healing tradition in a combined reprinting of two Ada Muir classics: *Healing Herbs of the Zodiac* and *Health and the Sun Signs: Cell Salts in Medicinal Astrology,* with an introduction by Master Herbalist and author Jude C. Williams.

Part one of this book covers the ills most often found in each zodiacal sign, along with the herbs attributed to healing those ills.

Part two covers the special mineral or cell salt needs of each sign. Cell salts, contained in fruits and vegetables, are necessary for the healthy activity of the human body.

In her introduction, Jude C. Williams increases the practical use of this book by outlining the basics of harvesting herbs and preparing tinctures, salves, and teas.
0-87542-575-5, 192 pgs., mass market, illus. $3.⁹⁹

THE JOY OF HEALTH
A Doctor's Guide to Nutrition and Alternative Medicine
by Zoltan P. Rona M.D., M.Sc.

Finally, a medical doctor objectively explores the benefits and pitfalls of alternative health care, based on exceptional nutritional scholarship, long clinical practice, and wide-ranging interactions with established and alternative practitioners throughout North America.

The Joy of Health is a must read before you seek the advice of an alternative health care provider. What are viable alternatives to standard cancer care? Is candida a real disease? Might hidden food allergies be the root of many physical and emotional problems?

- Get clear answers to commonly asked questions about nutrition and preventive medicine
- Explore various treatments for 47 conditions and diseases
- Make informed choices about food, diets, and supplements
- Explore 20 different types of diets and recipes
- Cut through advertising claims and vested-interest scare tactics
- Empower yourself to achieve a high level of wellness

0-87542-684-0, 264 pgs., 6 x 9, softcover $12.⁹⁵

THE COMPLETE HANDBOOK OF NATURAL HEALING
by Marcia Starck

Got an itch that won't go away? Want a massage but don't know the difference between rolfing, Reichian therapy, and reflexology? Tired of going to the family doctor for minor illnesses that you know you could treat at home—if you just knew how?

Designed to function as a home reference guide (yet enjoyable and interesting enough to be read straight through), this book addresses all natural healing modalities in use today: dietary regimes, nutritional supplements, cleansing and detoxification, vitamins and minerals, herbology, homeopathic medicine and cell salts, traditional Chinese medicine, Ayurvedic medicine, body work therapies, exercise, mental and spiritual therapies, and more. In addition, a section of 41 specific ailments outlines natural treatments for everything from acne to varicose veins.

0-87542-742-1, 416 pgs., 6 x 9 , softcover $12.⁹⁵